PLEASE RETURN
THANKS —

**BASED ON THE GREATEST SCIENTIFIC
DISCOVERY OF OUR CENTURY—A DIET
THAT GIVES YOU DRAMATICALLY
EXTENDED AND RENEWED YOUTH!**

Would you like to look into the mirror and
see your wrinkles faded, your body more erect
and bursting with energy, and other signs of
aging seemingly slowed down or erased?

Would you like to accomplish this in a matter
of weeks, simply by adding a few simple, in-
expensive, and tasty foods to your diet—without drugs, cosmetic surgery, or any other unnatural process?

Now at last it is possible, by following the
amazing diet based on the discovery of the
double helix, developed and successfully pa-
tient-tested by a practicing physician.

Dr. Frank's No-Aging Diet

The diet that puts to use our new scientific
knowledge of the aging process. Countless
thousands have already tried it. Don't wait too
long to try it yourself.

DR. BENJAMIN S. FRANK, now in private practice in New York City, is the author of *A New Approach to Degenerative Disease and Aging* and *Nucleic Acid Therapy of Aging and Degenerative Disease.*

Philip Miele, Professor of Communication Arts, New York Institute of Technology, is a longtime consultant in public relations.

Dr. Frank's No-Aging Diet

Benjamin S. Frank, M.D.
with
Philip Miele

A DELL BOOK

To Ruth Aley, literary agent, and Joyce Engelson, editor, the author and writer dedicate this book with awe and affection.

Published by
DELL PUBLISHING CO., INC.
1 Dag Hammarskjold Plaza
New York, N.Y. 10017

Dell books are available at discounts in quantity lots for sales promotion, industrial, or fund-raising use. Special books can also be created for the specific needs of any business.

For details contact the Special Marketing Division, Dell Publishing Co., Inc., 1 Dag Hammarskjold Plaza, New York, N.Y. 10017

Contents

PREFACE BY
SHELDON S. HENDLER, PH.D.

"Energy is the only life and is from the Body . . .
Energy is Eternal Delight."
—William Blake,
The Marriage of Heaven and Hell

Energy plays the major role in our lives. Political power struggles are directly related to who controls the energy sources of the world, whether it be oil to fuel our cars and heat our homes, or sugar and wheat to fuel our bodies. On a more personal level, we talk about our state of well-being in terms of how much energy we have available. When we are depressed we feel we have no energy and it is hard to do anything. We feel old and lifeless. When we are happy we have enough energy to move mountains. In the last several years there has been an exciting development of interest in ways to help us feel more energetic and to live life to the fullest. Notable among these ways are the bioenergetics movement, Yoga, transcendental meditation, exercise, massage, the Alexander technique, group therapy, and nutrition. It is to this last way—nutrition—that the present book is devoted.

I first met Dr. Benjamin Frank in the early 1960s, at which time I was pursuing my doctorate in biochemistry at Columbia University. My research interest at that time, as it has been ever since, was concerned with nucleic acids. In the early 1960s the excitement over nucleic acids was at its greatest heights. There was no question that at least some of the profound secrets of life could be gleaned by understanding the mysteries written within the nucleic acids. I will never forget the excitement, the wonder, the awe I felt when I first isolated DNA in my laboratory. As the DNA wound around my stirring rod in the test tube, I felt extremely close to the god—energy. Dr. Frank's enthusiasm about these magical molecules has never ceased. He felt from our earliest discussions about them that they undoubtedly must also be an elixir which when eaten could help people live more fulfilled lives. It is with just this great love that Dr. Frank has been treating his patients for as long as we have known each other. We have already seen that the building blocks of nucleic acids are involved in the production of the energy of life. It makes sense that diets rich in nucleic acids will increase the energy content of our cells. Some of Dr. Frank's successes could be attributed to an increase in energy.

It is said that we look as young as we feel. In this sense anything that makes us feel energetic will keep us young, if not in body, then surely in spirit. That is what Blake meant when he said "Energy is Eternal Delight." Dr. Frank's results with diets rich in nucleic acids suggest that these molecules contribute to the storehouse of energy of all our cells. More energy available to our brain cells should make us feel brighter. More energy available to all our cells should make us more resistant to many diseases. We certainly know that children who are malnourished have a tremendously decreased resistance to disease.

The current approach in most medical schools emphasizes the dietary importance of carbohydrates, fats and proteins for the fulfillment of our energy requirements. In the United States future doctors are taught that the daily intake of these three major components should include 40 percent carbohydrate, 40 percent fat and 20 percent protein. The importance of vitamins and minerals is also stressed.

It is accepted that by a series of biochemical reactions, the carbohydrates, fats and proteins are first broken down to their basic building blocks (glucose, fructose and galactose from the carbohydrates, fatty acids and glycerol from the fats, and amino acids from the proteins) in the gastrointestinal tract by biological catalysts known as the digestive enzymes. The basic build-

ing blocks are transported across the wall of the small
intestine into the blood and lymph systems of the body.
Ultimately the building blocks are transported into the
cells, which are the fundamental units of life of our
body. There, by another series of intricate biochemical
reactions known as intermediary metabolism, they produce the fundamental fuel of life. This is a molecule
called adenosine triphosphate or, more simply, ATP.
Vitamins and minerals are crucial to the process. It is
this molecule, ATP, which we need in order to write a
poem, throw a ball, make love, feel alive. The face and
body of an infant who is deprived of the dietary components necessary to make ATP often appears to be the
face and body of an old person.

However, it may be asked whether we get enough energy from just the traditionally accepted nutrients. It
happens that among the digestive enzymes there is in
the small intestine a group known as nucleases. These
enzymes break down crucial molecules called nucleic
acids into their basic building blocks, the nucleotides.
Without nucleic acids life as we know it could not have
developed. There are two major types of nucleic acids.
The genes of our cells, which determine all of our he-
reditary characteristics, contain the nucleic acid called
deoxyribonucleic acid or DNA. The other type, which
is involved in the actualization of the program of DNA,
is ribonucleic acid or RNA. DNA itself was discovered
in 1869 by Friedrich Miescher and RNA years later.
But it was not until the early 1950s that the roles of
these molecules began to be elucidated.

The building blocks of nucleic acids, the nucleotides,
besides forming these molecules, are involved in one
way or another in most of the chemical reactions within
our cells. ATP, the fuel of life, is itself a nucleotide.
Many of the vitamins, such as thiamine (B_1), ribo-
flavin (B_2), niacin (B_3), and pantothenic acid, work as
partner molecules with nucleotides to produce biological energy. Nucleotides play a major role in the production of carbohydrates, fats, proteins and, of course, nu-

cleic acids. Indeed, just as every work of art has a motif that gives it its shape as well as a reason for being, we can say that the chemical motif of life is the nucleotides.

Although the importance of nucleic acids in biological processes has been recognized for some time, the dietary importance of these molecules has only rarely been considered. The reason for this is quite simple. We know that the basic building blocks of nucleic acids, the nucleotides, can be synthesized from other nutrients, namely carbohydrates and proteins. However, the presence of certain biological processes may lead us to re-evaluate their dietary role. As was mentioned before, digestive enzymes do exist in the gastrointestinal tract for the conversion of nucleic acids into nucleotides. Furthermore, there are biosynthetic pathways within our cells for the conversion of components of the nucleotides, the so-called nucleotide bases, into the nucleic acid building blocks. It is of interest to point out that a deficiency in one of these pathways produces mental retardation. Therefore, we may infer from these biological findings that there is not a sufficient amount of nucleotides produced in the biochemical routes that make them from the other dietary components, and that indeed we require in our diets nucleic acids or their building blocks. *I know of no other medical person or nutritionist who has continuously stressed the dietary importance of nucleic acids as has Dr. Benjamin Frank.*

Only time and continued investigation will determine the ultimate scientific validity of Dr. Frank's claims, but in any event, this book is a significant landmark in the history of nutrition. For in introducing the subject of nucleic acids, he has opened the doors—to the general public—to the substances which form the very essence of life in a way that is edible, tasty, and very easily digested.

Sheldon S. Hendler, Ph.D.
Chairman, Division of Basic Sciences,
University of Baja California

1

Some Walking Miracles

Good health is the natural state of the human body. I believe in maintaining this state—and in restoring it if it is lost—in ways that are natural to the body: not with powerful drugs but with natural nutrients. I have found that these nutrients work better and are far safer than medicines which are so powerful (the word really should be dangerous) that the public must be protected from them by laws that require prescriptions.

Of course, everyone agrees that good nutrition is essential to good health. However, my research shows that it can be far more effective than was ever suspected, not only in maintaining good health but in restoring it when disease sets in. The no-aging diet outlined later will do this for you.

What has all this to do with aging? As soon as we are born, we begin to age, you might say. True, but as you will see, the older we grow the more susceptible we become to diseases, and diseases in turn speed up aging. What's more, these diseases spring from the same root cause. Treat the root cause of one and you are treating the root cause of the others.

This is a vastly different approach to health than you are accustomed to, so I will explain in more detail as simply as I can in later chapters. For the moment I will simply say that foods rich in DNA and RNA—nucleic acids—are the key. They are not strange foods; you probably eat them anyway, but not enough of them. They work wonders. My patients look younger and feel

younger by being healthy. They range in age from teen-
agers to men and women well into their eighties.

Let's take a look at some of my patients who have
benefited from nucleic-acid therapy. These are not
carefully selected cases, a few out of hundreds of thousands. They are patients who are part of the modest
practice of a single practicing physician.

When you read about their treatment you will notice
that some were given nucleic acid extracts as well as the
nucleic-acid-rich diet. These extracts, like the foods in
the diet, are natural substances but have been concentrated from yeast. They work on the same principles as
the diet, but they are stronger. You can buy them in tablet form at health food stores, but because they are
stronger they must be used under supervision of a physician who can take such necessary precautions as seeing
that the urine does not become too acid.

You can expect similar though less speedy results
from the diet. What is more, the diet is safe because it is
properly balanced for the vast majority of us.

One of the most interesting patients is medically typical: a 78-year-old licensed pilot who used to be older
than he is today. When he was 71 years old, Edward W.
Stitt was bald, arthritic, and suffering from failing eyesight, a painful case of diverticulitis, and chronic fatigue. Five years later on a mild winter's day he tarred
the hundred-fifty-foot roof of his workshop where he
upholsters antique automobiles in Lancaster, Pennsyl-
vania. The next day he rose at four A.M. to drive to
New York for one of the three or four checkups he now
has each year in my office. He walks with an almost
military snap, speaks crisply, to the point, and looks like
a vigorous man in his mid-fifties.

To the consternation of flight surgeons who have
tested his eyesight for renewal of his pilot's medical cer-
tificate, he reads telephone directories and other fine
print without glasses. His arthritis and diverticulitis
have completely disappeared and there is a thin growth
of hair on his once-bald head. "The truth is," he says,

"I'm younger now than I was five and ten years ago."

His treatment consisted of the nucleic-acid-rich diet, vitamins, and nucleic acid extracts. No aspirin or pain killers, no hormones, no drugs. The diet is not a list of fun-killing *don't*s but a regime of nourishing foods, largely fish and legumes. For Mr. Stitt, however, there is one *don't* which he cheerfully ignores: He still enjoys two dry Manhattans a day. "The only thing I don't like about the diet," he complains, "is that extra water I have to drink."

Hundreds of women and men like Mr. Stitt have been dramatically de-aged and have been partially or entirely freed from a variety of ills such as emphysema, heart disease, diabetic complications, arthritis, fading eyesight, loss of memory, plus a melancholy list of other debilitations of old age. (Also, as you will see later, one condition more associated with youth than old age—acne—is often dramatically relieved by nucleic-acid therapy.)

The important thing to note is that these conditions were not treated specifically or one at a time, as they would be in more conventional practice. The entire body was treated with nutrients fundamental to the body's basic processes.

At this point you may wonder why, as spectacular as the results were for Mr. Stitt, we mention him at all since he took special nucleic acid extracts along with the diet. Are these necessary and, if so, what role does the diet play?

The answer is that I am able to watch closely over my patients to see that complications do not set in. This means that I can give them far larger, more powerful doses of nucleic acid than I would recommend in a book for general readers. I do not know your state of health and must therefore limit my advice to you to a safe diet.

This should accomplish all that I say it does, only more slowly than if it were accompanied by the special extracts. The diet and the extracts work on the same principle; the extracts are more powerful.

The diet alone, without the more powerful extracts, has produced notable results. In a study which I conducted fifteen years ago, I put sixteen patients on the diet. They ranged in age from 25 to 60. Twelve of them were not told what to expect so they would not later report benefits simply because they were expecting them. All were ill, suffering from one degenerative disease or another.

A week to ten days later every one of them reported an increase in energy, a sense of well-being. They climbed stairs with less breathlessness and less fatigue. They continued to improve for a month or more. Then they were taken off the diet. They ate "normally"— good nourishing food but not the nucleic-acid-rich diet. In a month or two energy declined, fatigue returned, proving that what are widely considered normal, healthy diets are not enough to sustain good health.

One member of this group was a 49-year-old man who suffered from a painful heart condition, angina pectoris. Just a slow walk of a few hundred feet would cause almost paralyzing chest pains, and he would have to stop until they subsided. Now, with treatment combining the diet with nucleic acid extracts, he walks a mile or more with no discomfort. When pain does occur, it is brief and far less severe.

The diet, or the diet plus the extracts, leads to striking visible changes in the elderly. They begin to feel and look better in about a week. Their skin, once dry and sallow, looks moist and healthy. In about a month the skin tightens. Pinch the backs of their hands and the skin snaps back sooner. Deep lines and wrinkles begin to grow shallower, starting with the wrinkles of the forehead, followed by the lines from the nostrils to the mouth, and still later by the "crow's-feet" at the eye corners. Three or four months later the backs of the hands and the elbows become smoother. In short, they feel younger and look younger.

How much younger they look is, of course, subjective. The older the person, the more dramatically the appearance is changed. At 70 or 80 (judging by appearance alone), age seems to regress ten to fifteen years; at 60, about ten years; and at 30 to 50, five years or more.

Let us emphasize again: These changes in appearance are not just skin-deep. From a medical point of view they are not cosmetic at all. They stem from deep-down improvements in health.

2
A Revolution in the Making

Revolutions have a lot in common, whether they happen in astronomy, physics, medicine, or politics. Those who introduce a new idea pay dearly for their insolence, sometimes with their lives, often with ridicule, hardly ever without shattered reputations. Once the trauma of deep change is comfortably past we look back and wonder at the fuss people made over what appears now to be solidly based sweet logic. Who among us, if he had lived in the fifteenth century, would not have scoffed at a man who claimed the world was round? Even after he proved it? Or, more recently, that airplanes can fly, that germs can cause disease, that it is not evil to anesthetize patients when you operate on them?

To be honest, all of us might have been among the scoffers. Ideas are powerful; they structure our lives, and an elemental wisdom tells us that to accept a major new idea is to face major, unforeseen consequences. Let us not be too harsh with the scoffers. All change is not good, all truth not beautiful, all "progress" not improvement.

This must be said now because we are—at this moment—on the eve of a revolution in medical thought. The decorum of scientific discourse may be disturbed, some reputations may be endangered and, most important, some reputations may be endangered and, most important, the consequences are not entirely foreseeable however exciting the possibilities might be.

The stakes, for those who participate in it, will be high indeed. And when the barricades go up there will be honorable, competent people of goodwill as well as crackpots and knaves on both sides. Theory will be pitted against theory, one man's findings will be contradicted by another's, and the life's work of many a fine scientist will fall from the edge of his flat world.

This is a prerevolutionary moment in the world of medicine, not because of medicine's failures but because of its successes. The fundamental need today is not only for new ways of putting basic knowledge to work but also for new knowledge. A new and better drug for treating diabetes will be welcome, of course. But that would stem from what we already know about diabetes—that it is caused by a poorly functioning pancreas. More welcome, in fact more urgently needed, is new knowledge about why the pancreas does not work and what can be done to make it work.

Even this kind of knowledge is not fundamental enough to add up to the kind of revolution now in prospect. The next big step will be the kind of knowledge that will treat the human body as a whole, so that what we do to help one part of it at least does not injure another part, and at best helps it.

We are speaking of a unified theory of degenerative disease! It is coming.

I now offer such a new approach. It is a theory which explains such apparently diverse phenomena as aging, cataracts, heart disease, diabetes—and yes, even cancer in a single, unified way. There are findings to support the theory. I will tell you about them. Most important, I will tell you how you can benefit—safely—right now from these findings, even if the theory should later be proved wrong. That is the way with theories; even wrong or inadequate ones can lead to useful findings. The idea that the earth is the center of the universe, wrong as it is (and difficult as it was to change) nevertheless permitted development of accurate calendars.

You will be able to benefit from this theory in many ways without waiting for the world of science to adopt or reject it. By following a very safe and simple diet, you will start to feel better. Then, as if some strange miracle were taking place, you may start to look younger. Why do we say *may* start to look younger? Does this word cover some hidden doubts?

No, the diet works. No doubt about that. But you may already be in superb health, may look young for your age. In this case, the diet will probably not make you look younger. For you, the diet will be a powerful preventive measure—delaying the inevitable onset of age, helping to guard against the onset of degenerative diseases.

For others, in fact for most American adults, the diet will smooth away wrinkles on the face, neck, and hands as it lessens or even reverses the ravages of the degenerative diseases which, taken together, are what old age is. Your skin will become tighter and glow with health.

Here's how it happens: Our bodies are made up of cells—thousands of billions of them. They are born, they reproduce themselves, they age, they die. In reproducing they make copies of themselves. As we age, these copies differ from their predecessors in various ways, each way being a disease in itself. In other words, old age is like a collection of degenerative diseases: muscle atrophy, arthritis, cataracts, heart disease, diabetes, cancer, emphysema—all afflictions which strike as we grow older.

Today, we tend to attack each of these diseases separately, often in ways which create wear and tear on the body and even trigger other diseases. Consider that the drugs most often used to treat serious diseases are available only on prescription. That's because these drugs have side effects. If they were safe as milk there would be no need for prescriptions. Lifesaving medicines can be hazardous to our health, yet as we grow older we must depend more and more on them.

Because these diseases have different symptoms, conventional medicine finds it reasonable to treat them differently. But my research shows that they have the same underlying causes, and it points to a way of treating them all together with a single, natural approach. I believe they can be treated by cooperating with the body's own processes instead of insulting it with powerful substances which are foreign to it.

Back to the cells: Among other things, they are made up of various kinds of nucleic acids. Two of these are in charge of what happens—RNA (ribonucleic acid) and DNA (deoxyribonucleic acid). Working together, they are fundamental to the life process itself. DNA in the nucleus tells RNA on the periphery what to do. Good high-quality DNA—the kind in young, healthy bodies—issues precise instructions on what kind of cells to form and where. High-quality RNA—once again the kind in young, healthy bodies—does precisely what it is told to do.

But the quality of these nucleic acids deteriorates as we age. They create faulty cells which in turn create more faulty cells in ways which add up to degenerative diseases.

Here now is the heart of the new theory: There are natural direct and indirect sources of high-quality DNA and RNA which can be supplied from outside the body to nourish our cells and return them all to a healthy state. It is possible to keep doing this. This means it is possible to remain healthy far longer than the general experience of the human race. It means much-delayed old age.

Let's state this differently: It is possible, according to this theory, to remain healthy as long as you live and to live much longer.

Has this been proved yet? No.

Has it been disproved? No.

Is there evidence to support the theory? Yes. Plenty.

Then what more is needed? More evidence and more work to get even better nutrients (nucleic acids and other related nutrients from outside the body) to do the job.

If there is evidence to support the theory, how can it be proved wrong?

There is no question about the findings. Maybe, just maybe, the explanation for them, which is what any theory is all about, will turn out to be something else. I do not think so. This is what the scientific discourse, which has not started yet, will be all about. To start it, I have set forth the theory and related findings in scientific detail in a book for the medical profession, *Nucleic Acid Therapy of Aging and Degenerative Disease.**

Meanwhile, even before any controversy begins, and no matter how it turns out, you can begin to profit right now, safely and easily. You can slow down your aging process, maybe even grow a little younger, starting right now.

* Third ed., published in 1975 by Fiquima, Lisbon.

3
New Energy for Our Cells

All living things are made of cells—polar bears and boa constrictors, tomatoes and sharks, bats and bacteria, mice and men. What's more, the cells are strikingly similar—they have an undeniable family resemblance. Although, as we will see later, there are significant differences, let us look for a moment at the similarities. We will describe a typical cell, one which is as much like other cells as a typical cat is like all other cats.

Our typical cell is a globule, a tiny ball, so tiny it would take about three thousand of them placed side by side to measure an inch. Now, let's magnify it to the size of a grape. It has a skin or membrane to protect it. Even in plants this cellular skin is pretty much like ours. In all of us (snakes, bumblebees, you, and me) the cell's skin is made up of sugars, of proteins, and fatty materials called lipids. Like all living things, the cell requires nourishment and, alas, like everything that eats, it produces waste. The cell's skin is remarkably designed to let into the cell only things that are good for it and to let out of the cell only its wastes. Unhappily, this does not always work. Viruses, some poisons, radiation like cosmic rays from space and X rays, can enter and do their mischief by damaging the cell and causing it to reproduce in ways that add up to degenerative diseases and old age.

In the very center of the cell, about a quarter of the size of the cell itself, is the nucleus. This is the headquarters. Here information is stored about what the cell is supposed to do—whether, for example, it is supposed to be part of an eyelid or a liver. Every so often, depending on where it is, it will divide and become two cells, all on orders issued by the nucleus. If everything goes well, these two cells are identical to their predecessor. However, everything does not always go well because of the mischief we just mentioned caused by viruses, poisons, and radiation.

This nucleus contains, among other things, three important types of substances: enzymes, histones, and DNA. Enzymes are catalysts which speed up or make the going smoother for all life processes. Histones have something (not fully understood) to do with the cell's functions and reproduction. DNA is the master chemical, a giant molecule which makes up one of the nucleic acids. It regulates production of the enzymes and other proteins, and therefore plays the master role—perhaps solo, perhaps along with other agents—in determining what the cell's characteristics are and will be. In all cells of all living nature you will find this DNA, though not in the red blood cells of men and some other vertebrates.

Let's pause a moment to look more closely at this giant molecule which plays such a central role. Let us construct a model in our imagination. We need a tall, slim bottle, two pieces of ribbon, and a handful of toothpicks. Wrap a piece of ribbon around the bottle in a clockwise spiral. Do the same with the other piece of ribbon. Next, imagine that the ribbon will retain its shape as we remove the bottle and discard it. Now place the toothpicks between the ribbons as if they were the steps of a spiral staircase, about four to every complete turn of the two ribbons. There you have it.

The ribbon is made of sugar, deoxyribose, and a phosphate. The toothpicks are the purines and pyrimidines. All this, which makes up the DNA molecule, can be found in butterfly wings and human earlobes. *What's more*—this is the underpinning of the diet which will be explained later—*the DNA components found in one form of life can do their work on the cells of another!*

This does not mean that when you eat a peach its DNA will tell your cells to turn you into a peach. Instead, it will help get word to your cells telling them to do what they are supposed to do.

Back to our typical cell. So far we have looked at the skin and the tiny nucleus, or headquarters, in the center. Between the two is the area where the cell's work is done—the cytoplasm. We can think of it pretty much as if it were a factory—raw materials come in and are sorted, stored, and made into the cell's products; waste material is discarded.

Between this manufacturing area and headquarters there must be some form of communication. It works roughly as follows: The manufacturing area sends raw materials to the headquarters, where they are reassembled into a message or messenger. (They are one and the same, Marshall McLuhan will be pleased to know, making the medium the message.) This message-messenger is another nucleic acid, Messenger RNA. Once formed by the DNA in headquarters, this RNA leaves for the manufacturing area, where its orders are carried out. In the process it comes apart and its constituents become part of other processes. The RNA molecule is smaller than the DNA and the "ribbon" is made of a different kind of sugar, ribose.

All of us started as a single cell following an intimate moment in our parents' history. This cell divided into two, these into two again, and so on. How come some of them got together to form a liver and others to form a big toe? This is a question that teases the mind. We do not know.

Altogether the human body contains many trillion cells. Most of them reproduce themselves before they wear out. Some do not. Those in the heart muscles and nerves in the brain do not. All the others that do reproduce themselves have progeny of increasingly lower quality, which, as we have said, is what aging is all about. The reason, according to more of the theory we are about to describe, is that energy for production and

repair of DNA and RNA declines and what is produced is of lower quality. This, according to my theory,
results in a DNA which is providing poor instructions
because it too is deficient in quality. Brain and heart
DNA decay too.

This leads us to conclude that the way to maintain
health and to restore damaged health is to provide
energy-giving nutrients from outside the body. Among
the most essential nutrients are the nucleic acids, RNA
and DNA, which have received virtually no serious
medical attention and which are slowly, tragically disap-
pearing from our diets. In fact, with all the scientific
attention being focused on RNA and DNA, it is amazing that conventional medicine has ignored the dramatic
part they play in our diet.

We have just described the roles they play in our
cells. In addition, they are energy-ensuring nutrients.
They provide the kind of energy the cell needs to create
its own high-quality RNA and DNA and to repair the
body's damaged nucleic acids. A young cell can normally repair this damage because it has the needed energy. The older cell needs help to slow down or reverse
the aging process and combat the degenerative diseases
that are the unwelcome companions of old age. This is
what the diet will do.

If this seems spectacular, it is nothing compared with
what follows.

Let us look for what causes the slow deterioration of
the cell's ability to reproduce itself accurately and correct *that*. This is another way of saying let's look for the
underlying cause of aging and eliminate it! There is a
perfectly logical way to go about this.

First, let's find places in the body where cells do not
reproduce themselves at all. In the brain and in the
muscles at maturity, no new nerve and muscle cells are
created. Now, what is different about them? First, no
cancer grows in brain nerve cells and only rarely in
muscle cells. (So-called brain cancer is really in the in-
terconnecting cells, not the nerve tissue of the brain it-

self.) Second, brain and muscle have extra-high energy needs. For example, the brain itself is only 2 percent of the body's weight, yet it uses 20 percent of all the oxygen used by the body at rest.

Now, put these facts together with one more: Cancer cells do not use much oxygen. In other words, where our cells use oxygen the most, cancer is least likely to occur.

Before we look into what this means, let's answer a question which may have occurred to you: If muscle cells do not reproduce, how come our muscles get bigger and harder when we use them? How can they increase in size without new cells being added? The answer is that the cells grow; they do not increase in number.

Back now to this subject of energy needs. For our cells to reproduce and do all the work they do in our bodies, two things are needed: raw materials and energy. This is life in action. Everything we do, everything we think, uses energy and raw materials. Eating, drinking, and breathing are the ways we get the necessary raw materials. Chemical processes which are immensely complex break these chemicals down to free energy for use in the processes themselves and to create other chemicals useful to our bodies. So much energy is involved that if this were to take place at once we would explode. Happily, our biochemical processes are divided into steps, each carefully directed by enzymes with the assistance of coenzymes. Altogether they make up what we call metabolism.

One chemical process is central to all others: a metabolic process which provides the energy for the other metabolic systems. It takes place inside the factory part of the cell and is called the Krebs cycle—sometimes the citric-acid cycle. It is the same in all animal life and almost the same in plant life. It is a nine-step oxidative cycle—"oxidative," of course, because oxygen plays a vital role in it.

This cycle creates hydrogen electrons by breaking

down compounds which come from our foods. These electrons leave the cycle at several points and are carried, by a sort of bucket brigade, along electron transport chains. As they travel along these chains their energy becomes part of the structure of one of the most important molecules in our bodies, ATP (adenosine triphosphate). It is the primary energy carrier of our cells.

If any link in the electron transport chain becomes damaged, all the others are weakened. My research on nucleic acids and other research on low-tryptophane diets in the United States have led me to a theory that this chain becomes damaged in two ways, both of them perfectly "normal." The results pile up; we age.

In simplified, very simplified terms, here is one of the two ways I believe this happens: When we eat proteins they are broken down into more simple chemicals needed by the body and into waste products. One of these chemicals is a by-product of tryptophane. It has no business in the electron transport chain but, because it fits neatly into it, enters as an unwanted substitute for a certain coenzyme (coenzyme Q). The cells, noting that this coenzyme is not at work, produce less of it. Meanwhile, its stand-in is messing up the vital electron transport chain by failing to do the coenzyme's job: transferring energy from sugar (glucose) to the body's main energy-storing molecule, ATP. Instead, the energy never enters the cells and is wasted.

Thus the power needed for all the cell's functions is reduced. Defects in the outer and inner membranes of the cells—membranes that are critical in controlling the cell's responses to hormones and other substances—arise in this way. All this is "normal"—it takes place routinely in all of us, causing a slow loss of energy and reduced cell efficiency and self-repair, leading to roughly predictable life spans in the various animal species. The greater the metabolic rate, the shorter the life span. In this way we are built to "self-destruct," to die ultimately of old age and its complications. The phrase "natural causes" once used on death certificates is not too wide of the mark.

This suggests three ways of fighting harmful tryptophane derivatives: One, give the body more of the natural materials it normally uses to make coenzyme Q and other parts of the electron transport chain; two, give the body more raw materials for making ATP, thus invigorating the electron transport chain; three (which has not yet been accomplished), discover how to prevent tryptophane from producing the by-product which interferes with coenzyme Q. The no-aging diet accomplishes the first two.

Since tryptophane's mischief is a factor which limits the natural life span of different animal species, the life spans can be stretched by weakening tryptophane's effect. Other researchers have already learned that laboratory rats live longer and in better health on diets lower in protein and calories, and also low in tryptophane. Humans too live longer on relatively low-protein and low-calorie diets. However, proteins are essential nutrients and therefore if we rely on diet alone some tryptophane breakdown in the wrong way is inevitable.

When a way is found not just to undo the negative work of tryptophane but to prevent it from working at all, and to do the same with other similar degenerative processes that may be found in the electron transport chain, it will be entirely possible to prolong human life, with youthful vigor, not by decades but by centuries. Now, sadly, we can speak only of decades since we are limited to the new ways of nourishing the body with the raw materials of coenzyme Q and ATP, and possibly by some other electron transport chain molecules or their precursors.

We mentioned earlier that the Krebs cycle becomes damaged in two ways. The second way occurs outside the cycle. In processing sugar, a series of steps takes place before the Krebs cycle begins. These steps do not use oxygen. The connection between them and the

Krebs cycle, a key energy-transfer point, allows just enough energy to keep the cycle going at whatever rate is necessary. It is a sort of gateway made of enzymes. When somehow the gateway is clogged, the energy stays in the non-oxygen-using phase, slowing down the Krebs cycle and at the same time helping to create the kind of cells that do not need much oxygen—cancer (and perhaps many other degenerative diseases). In other words, I see cancer as a metabolic disorder. Getting the non-oxygen-using steps properly linked up again with the Krebs cycle, among other related things, is the way to help defeat cancer, to prevent it, to cure it once it occurs. I have done this with mice.

In laboratory mice with cancer (sarcoma 180 and other tumors) the connecting gateway was opened by injections of nucleic-acid-related nutrients plus other nutrient vitamins important for the functioning of the gateway enzyme. It worked. Tumors stopped growing, became smaller, then died. The mice lived on.

A word of caution. The no-aging diet will improve general health and retard aging. It will not cure cancer. It remains to be proved that what happened in the lucky laboratory mice can be made to happen in humans. What is more, the materials used in the mice may not be the very best, the fastest-acting, or the most potent materials available. More research needs to be done, though the basis has been laid.

As we can see, fairly high Krebs-cycle and electron-chain activity is antiaging, anti-degenerative disease, anticancer. However, where this high-energy cycle works at its peak, in the brain and muscles, no cancer cells are formed and neither are healthy new cells formed. Brain damage is tragically final. It is interesting to speculate on the possibility of carefully narrowing the gateway to the high-energy cycle to produce growth (not cancer) to create brain cells when needed and thus repair damage from strokes, arteriosclerosis, multiple sclerosis, and Parkinson's disease, and to restore the mental keenness often dulled with age.

More to the point, I have proved that—working on my theory that the basic cause of aging is the loss of energy to the cell and that this loss of energy is caused by interference with the Krebs cycle and the connecting energy-transport chain—the aging process can be slowed down.

Nucleic acids in the diet increase ATP production and step up the energy of the electron transport chain, even after some parts of it are damaged. This energy repairs damage in old cells, causing them to function like younger ones. I have shown this antiaging effect of nucleic acids time and again with hundreds of my patients.

I am far from being the only medical researcher, or the first, to be interested in nucleic acids. DNA was discovered long ago, in 1869, and RNA many years later. Though it was not until the early 1950s that the role of these molecules really began to be understood and explained, many scientists have since done spectacular work studying nucleic acids and diseases. (Much of the cancer research now in progress is focused on DNA's role in designing living cells.)

In Europe, organ-specific tissues (which contain nucleic acids) in injectable form are widely used. These are taken from specific organs of unborn animals and injected into humans for the repair of the corresponding organ.

My work is different in several respects. I aim at improving the health of the entire body rather than one organ or one disease at a time; my therapy involves both RNA and sometimes DNA; my patients take them orally, as in the diet, not by injection; and I regard nucleic acids not as medicines but as natural nutrients.

4

The
No-Aging
Diet

What you are about to read will probably come as a surprise to you. This no-aging diet tells you *what to eat, not what not to eat* like most diets. Of the twenty-one meals we eat each week, the diet involves only eight or ten. The goods are easy to find—in fact they are on most restaurant menus. You are probably accustomed to most of them. The biggest change the diet will bring will not be in your eating habits but in your health.

The diet consists of a variety of foods rich in nucleic acids, plus fluids and vitamins. They are spread throughout the week in a way that will provide a daily intake of one or two grams of nucleic acids in dietary form. Do not settle for the same dosage in extracts, which you may find in tablet form. These do not contain all the nutrients of real food and they require medical supervision.

Here are the rules:

1. Four days a week, eat a three- or four-ounce can of small sardines. To avoid weight gain, drain off any oil they may be packed in.

2. One other day a week, have salmon (canned or fresh) as a main course.

3. On still another day, have shrimp, lobster, squid, clams, or oysters as a main course.

4. On the remaining day, eat any other kind of fish as a main course.

In other words, you must have seafood seven times a

week—sardines four times, salmon once, nonvertebrate seafood once, and any kind of fish once.

5. Eat calves' liver once a week.

6. Once or twice a week have beets, beet juice or borscht.

7. Once or twice a week have a side dish of lentils, peas, lima beans, or soybeans.

8. Each day eat at least one of the following: asparagus, radishes, onions, scallions, mushrooms, spinach, cauliflower, or celery.

9. Each day take one strong multivitamin after any meal. (When you buy them, ask for therapeutic strength.)

10. Each day, drink two glasses of milk, preferably skimmed.

11. Each day, drink a glass of fruit or vegetable juice.

12. Each day, drink at least four glasses of water—more in the summer to replace perspiration.

You can fall off the diet once in a while with no great harm. However, never neglect items 10, 11, 12. This is the only strict part of the diet. If you do not have these fluids, your urine may become acid and cause complications if you are one of the small number of people with high blood uric-acid levels. The chief complications are kidney stones and gout. If you are conscientious about the fluids, there's no reason to worry about kidney stones resulting from these foods.

If you are familiar with gout, you may know that many, in fact most, of the foods listed above are precisely the ones gout sufferers are told to avoid. Strangely, however, this diet can be used as an effective part of the treatment in gout, provided it is under close medical supervision to keep down the uric acid.

Another word of warning: If you are under a doctor's care, follow his advice. This book does not know you; your doctor does. This is particularly true if you are on another diet.

There are no firm *don't*s to this diet, but to be on the safe side I would avoid foods that are chemically grown and prepared. Chemical fertilizer use depletes the soil of trace minerals which are vital to health. Other chemicals used in food preparation are not natural to the body and may be harmful. Besides, organically grown foods taste better.

I would avoid muscle meats too (steaks, chops, roasts) and dairy fats; they are high in saturated fats and may raise your cholesterol level too high. Milk is important but I recommend fat-free (skimmed) milk.

Sugar and starches also raise blood fat levels and may lead to overweight, so I would go easy on these.

Alcohol should be avoided too. Cocktails and beer and wine with meals tend to raise uric-acid levels. It is to prevent this that the diet places such heavy emphasis on fluids.

Salt and other seasonings should be used sparingly for related reasons.

If there is anything in this diet you particularly do not like, it is possible to make substitutions. If, for example, you simply hate sardines or liver, you may substitute another nucleic-rich food. The table of nucleic-acid-rich foods on page 81 will help you.

Perhaps more helpful to you will be the recipes. Since our diets are becoming poorer and poorer in nucleic acids, we are less and less exposed to imaginative ways of preparing foods rich in them. If you think you do not like sardines, keep your mind open until you try several of the ways of preparing them.

Sardines, you will notice, are particularly rich in nucleic acids. They contain ½ to 1 percent nucleic acid, while liver has up to ½ percent and muscle meats like steak have only 1/20 of one percent. However, nucleic acids do not work alone. Obviously there are other nutrients the body needs. Sardines, as well as other fish from the sea, are rich in other things such as essential oils and minerals which are not as abundant in land-based foods. One of these minerals, vanadium, also helps to lower blood cholesterol. Sardines and other fish have practically no cholesterol.

Nonvertebrate seafoods are also rich in nucleic acids, though they contain large quantities of cholesterol. Medical opinion about the dangers of cholesterol in foods is divided, so if you have a heart condition or high blood pressure it is better to play it safe and avoid lobsters, clams, shrimp, oysters and crabs. A healthy person should have no trouble with these nourishing foods, but so many of us have bodies so degenerated by years of improper diet and pollution that even when good natural foods are eaten, they cannot be properly metabolized until the body has time to repair itself.

Incidentally, you may wonder why some foods are richer in nucleic acids than others—why, for instance, sardines contain more than tuna, why salmon too contains slightly more than tuna and fish in general. I have often wondered about this too and must accept it, for the time being at least, as one of nature's secrets.

When you have been on this diet for a few months, your body will begin metabolizing fats more efficiently, and it will be safer to make substitutions without fear of cholesterol content.

Meanwhile, you will find a spectacular improvement in your health by returning for your nourishment to the sea, where all life began. It is entirely possible to follow another diet while you follow this one. For example, if you are on a weight-reducing diet, a salt-free diet, or a diabetic diet, you will probably find this one compatible. Your doctor will know.

A word now about vitamins. Medical science has known of the existence of vitamins for most of this century. Certain diseases, like beriberi, scurvy, pellagra, are well known to be caused by vitamin deficiencies.

How can it be, you might ask, that there is still so much controversy about how much we need of which vitamins to stay healthy? Ask the average American physician whether you should take vitamin supplements and he will probably say, "Fine, if you want more expensive urine." The truth is, he's perfectly right if all you do is take vitamins combined with the usual American diet of chemically grown vegetables, hot dogs, hamburgers, or steak and soft drinks.

Vitamins, like nucleic acids, do not work alone; hence the confused medical reports we have all been reading.

You remember, for example, that Dr. Linus Pauling said that very large doses of vitamin C could be a cure for the common cold.

Then about five years later came word from a researcher of the U.S. Public Health Service that large vitamin C doses reduced sick days among a group of Navajo children by some thirty percent.

More recently a far-reaching Canadian study showed that patients who take large doses at the beginning of colds recover faster but that the vitamin was of little use in preventing colds.

Still more recently, an article in the *Journal of the American Medical Association* said that a detailed scrutiny of all published studies for the past thirty-five years failed to prove the value of large vitamin C doses.

Meanwhile the Food and Drug Administration says we can get along quite nicely on a tenth or a twentieth of these large doses. Surely Dr. Pauling's evidence would support higher doses—though just how high is not yet clear.

There is a similar controversy regarding other vitamins. What are we to believe?

Are we simply paying for more expensive urine, or are we buying better health?

The answer is that it depends on what else we eat along with the vitamins. In my work on this diet, I have seen patient after patient show improvement on nucleic acids without vitamin supplements, but greater improvement with them. Vitamin supplements combined with the typical American diet have proved to be of very little use. Combine them, as in this nucleic acid diet, and the results add up to more youthful appearance, more vigor, and a fundamental improvement in health. The conclusion is unavoidable that nucleic acids are vitally essential nutrients.

5

It
Shows
on
Your Face

You do not have to go to medical school to read certain signs of health on the skin. We know that dry, wrinkled skin, particularly on the face, neck, and hands, is a telltale sign of age.

The nucleic acid diet can revolutionize the appearance of most Americans, because most of us are in poor health and aging faster than necessary.

What can you expect from the diet?

As mentioned in Chapter 1, if you are showing signs of aging, you will look younger as your health improves. Wrinkles of the forehead will smooth out. This will be noticeable in a month or two. Then the deep lines from the nostrils to the corners of the mouth (the parentheses of an aging face) will become shallower and the crow's-feet at the eye corners will begin to lighten. In a few months you may even look more youthful than you do in photographs taken a decade ago.

In about four months, the backs of your hands and elbows will be smoother. On the backs of your hands the skin will be tighter, as it was when you were younger. You will notice that calluses on your feet (which are often caused by poor circulation) may begin to disappear. This is particularly true of diabetics who are on nucleic-acid-rich diets.

Your skin will be moist and will glow with the color of good health. The whites of your eyes, if dulled with age, will begin to sparkle. All this in about four months with no drugs, no plastic surgery—just safe, wholesome foods which are tragically neglected in most American diets.

Strangely, while the diet will moisten the dry skin of the aging person, it will dry the oily skin of the young and at the same time relieve one of the most poignant afflictions of adolescents: acne.

I conducted a study of fourteen patients ranging in age from 19 to 31 who suffered from mild to moderately severe acne. They all showed visible signs of improvement after nucleic-acid therapy. All were advised to avoid fats, candies, soft drinks, and chocolate, as they had been doing before I put them on the diet. I gave no special instructions about face washing.

In two months improvement was apparent in all fourteen cases. In four months all signs of acne had disappeared from the faces of most of them.

Six women in this group complained that the nucleic-acid therapy did not prevent their acne from becoming worse while they were menstruating. The RNA dosage was doubled during these periods and the problem was eliminated.

The diet alone can be of immense help. One woman who read an article about it in the June 1974 issue of *Cosmopolitan* wrote:

> For the past eleven years I have suffered from acne. I have been to a total of seven different doctors, but nothing has ever really helped my bad complexion. Then I read the article called "The Youth Diet" by Philip Miele in your June issue, and for the first time in eleven years there was a very marked improvement in my skin. It is almost cleared up. I just cannot thank you enough for that article. My 65-year-old mother also went on the diet and is experiencing surprisingly wonderful results.

From the point of view of your appearance, what is particularly exciting about this diet is that you need not clog up your pores with cosmetics that nature never intended for your skin. And there is no need for plastic surgery, which is expensive and, in many cases, temporary. The diet is completely natural. What it does for you is not just skin-deep.

6

Helpful
Nutrition
for
Drug Addicts
and
Alcoholics

Sick people generally do not feel well. This sounds obvious to the point of being fatuous, but it is an insight that can lead to important help for the addict or alcoholic seeking to free himself from his sickness. Not feeling well can lead the addict to do the very thing that causes his illness. If we can make him feel well, in fact be well, we add to the crucial strength he needs for his struggle back to health.

The alcoholic, weakened from malnutrition and poor sleep, suffering from a hangover, cannot be expected to have the vigorous resolve needed for what amounts to a demanding battle for self-liberation. The same is true of the drug addict. Another drink, another fix, and all seems well for a little while longer. If we could provide him with a lasting sense of well-being, the psychological need for the drink or fix would be lessened. Not eliminated, but lessened, because, to say one more obvious thing, a healthy body permits the mind to enjoy good health too.

The alcoholic often suffers from malnutrition—particularly a deficiency of B vitamins. In advanced cases his nervous system may be severely damaged and his personality, even while sober, markedly changed. Cirrhosis of the liver is a well-known affliction of alcoholics.

I studied the usefulness of nucleic-acid therapy with twenty-four alcoholic patients—bloated, weakened men and women with trembling hands and sallow complexions. Eighteen of them had damaged livers, though not cirrhosis.

Immediately before I began their treatment, all had stopped drinking. Two weeks of intensive nourishment with nucleic-acid extracts and vitamins led to a sharp decrease in tremors, vastly improved complexions, increased strength, and a new sense of well-being. In about six weeks, all who had damaged livers showed signs of healing.

To the extent that good health and a sense of well-being make the road back from alcoholism easier, every patient in this study was helped. Whether it was enough help to permit each to win his personal battle against this addiction cannot be known, because follow-up observations were not possible.

Drug addiction, though not as widespread as alcoholism, is even more tragic. Mental dullness, inability to concentrate, malnutrition, skin infections, hepatitis, and in some cases lung, brain, and kidney abscesses are among the prices addicts pay. The road back is longer and far more difficult, and the treatment slightly different. While the alcoholic receives no alcohol as part of his treatment, the drug addict is often given a drug—methadone—in gradually reduced amounts.

In another study, I treated more than one hundred heroin addicts with nucleic-acid extracts, vitamins, and decreasing doses of methadone. The addicts ranged in age from 21 to 76 and had been addicts for one to ten years. Most were suffering from severe mental and physical deterioration. They were unkempt, unclean, and listless.

Results were dramatic; in one to two weeks they no longer looked haggard. Their strength had begun to return. For many, this new vitality was something they had not felt in years.

The third week there were encouraging signs of what a new sense of well-being can do for people who had so largely destroyed themselves. Most of them were able to accelerate the reduction of their methadone doses. They wore clean, pressed clothing and carried themselves with pride. About a third of them spoke of returning to work.

Some patients, however, did not fare as well. About 15 percent discontinued the nucleic-acid therapy but continued with methadone. The contrast between them and the 85 percent who remained on the program was stark.

While nucleic-acid therapy is no cure for alcoholism and drug addiction, it clearly helps repair damage caused by these diseases and strengthens victims for the torment they must face in returning to normal life.

7

Eat Your Way to Healthy Body Heat

From the steaming rain forests of Central Africa to the frozen wastes of the polar regions, the normal human body temperature is the same—98.6°F. Yet there are differences among those of us who live in the same climate.

Ever notice on a winter day that when most people are bundled up in heavy clothing, a few are dressed as if it were spring?

Not far from the Antarctic, on the freezing wind-beaten coast of Tierra del Fuego, the Indians who live there walk about almost naked. Of course, they are used to it, but there is more to it than that.

Why do some feel the cold more than others? It has to do with ATP, which, as we mentioned earlier, fuels almost all the body's metabolic reactions. These reactions give off heat. Nucleic acids cause production of ATP, and ATP powers the reactions that produce nucleic acids, a beautiful life-sustaining cycle—as long as it works. When it runs down or when something interferes with it, nucleic acids from outside the body can give it new life, keep it running at a healthy rate. This brings us back to the diet and why the Indians of Tierra del Fuego are so resistant to the cold.

They are not the beneficiaries of any special medical therapy. They live by the sea and eat what it provides: fish, which is central to their diet. Their fish, like all items in the no-aging diet, nourish their bodies with large quantities of nucleic acids which keep ATP production in high gear and thus help keep them warm.

You will notice that the diet will do the same for you though you may never run naked in Antarctic regions.

You may wonder how important this is compared with all the dramatic things the diet can do for us. We Americans live in warm houses and most of us are adequately clothed. Are we dealing here with an interesting but small side benefit of the diet?

No. Aside from keeping us more comfortable in winter there are other, very significant values to being able to maintain a steady body temperature. The easily chilled body is more vulnerable to infections. What's more, the person who is seriously chilled faces the danger of accidents because his alertness is impaired, his reaction time is slower, and he tires more easily. The swimmer with chattering teeth and blue lips may be overcome with dangerous fatigue and muscle cramps. The chilled skier or motorcyclist has lost that precious edge of instant judgment which can save his life. Benefits to the space program are obvious.

Since my theory sees the human body not as a machine but as a process, not as an assembly of parts but as a remarkably complex organization of interacting and therefore interdependent cycles, surprising relationships come to light between diseases which are widely believed to be different and distinct. I have already outlined this in an earlier chapter.

Since I became accustomed to this way of thinking I am less and less astonished when my search for interrelatedness leads to connections never made before. Just as I see an underlying common cause (and therefore prevention and remedy) for such apparently unconnected diseases as cataracts, heart disease, and emphysema, I can, relating the body to its "outside" environment, see a relationship between this diet and the quality of the air we breathe. The word *outside* is in quotations because nothing is totally separate or outside anything—everything exists in interaction with everything else.

The reasoning is simple, so simple that unless you become accustomed to this holistic method of thought it will sound foolish to you. If you eat foods that strengthen your body's ability to maintain its 98.6° temperature, you will live more comfortably in cooler homes. This means less fuel need be burned to heat our homes. Less fuel burning means cleaner air—not much cleaner, but a little. More important, heating dries the air in our homes. Less heating will help maintain a healthier level of moisture in the air.

This body-warming effect of the diet came to my attention by accident one winter night about fifteen years ago. I helped a dinner guest on with her coat, put on my own, and walked out onto a windy Manhattan corner for a taxi. While we waited I removed my coat; my guest snuggled for warmth in her heavy fur.

The next day my patients complained that my office was cold. Though I was usually more sensitive to the cold than others, I was sitting comfortably near an open window.

I felt fine but I took my temperature just in case. It was normal. My patients had normal temperatures too.

I had just run an experiment on myself with nucleic acids. Perhaps that was the cause. To find out, I tried the same experiment on two groups of rats. One group was given a nucleic-acid treatment, the other (for comparison) was not. Members of the first group slept far apart in their cage, the second group huddled together for warmth. Clearly one group required more heat from outside their bodies than the other.

Later, patients mentioned to me that after nucleic-acid therapy had begun they needed less heavy clothing in cold weather. One of these patients suffered from diabetes, which normally reduces tolerance to the cold. Then came a warning signal—a few of these patients, mostly those on very high dosages of extracts, said they were a little more uncomfortable in the heat than they had been before.

Back to the rats to see how they reacted to heat. The room temperature was boosted to 105°, then to 110°F.

The ones on nucleic acid extracts survived nicely; three of the eight in the comparison or control group died.

This experiment with the rats seemed to indicate that nucleic acids can actually protect against extreme heat as they do against extreme cold. I repeated the experiment several times with the same results, leading me to conclude that the slight discomfort in the heat experienced by a few of my patients was of no significance.

Edward Stitt, the 78-year-old licensed pilot, walking along New York streets in mid-November, carries his spring coat over his arm.

8

Eat Better; You'll Breathe Easier

Old people wheeze and cough more than young people do. They clear their throats before they speak and they run out of breath very quickly. This is "normal" for the aged. Their lungs are deteriorating.

Millions of Americans, mostly those well along in years, have emphysema. The symptoms are the same as those mentioned above, only worse, much worse. In advanced cases each breath can be an agony. What happens is that the lungs become enlarged, filled with air that can be expelled only with great effort.

If you do not have emphysema and wonder what it is like, try this: Take a deep breath. Now exhale just a little. Inhale again, and exhale just a little. Now cough, once again without exhaling very much. Now add pain and fatigue and you have some idea of what it is like. Remember you are sitting still reading a book. Try walking around like this for a few hours and you will get the idea more clearly.

If you are a smoker and do not have emphysema yet and would prefer not to have it, put your cigarette out and never light another. This will be the best way to prevent further damage. Despite all that has been learned about smoking, most of us are aware only of its gross effects. We know it may cause lung and heart disease. This is not enough to know. Smoking destroys nutrients in the body, reduces the body's ability to use efficiently those nutrients that remain, dulls the mind, and slows us down. What it accelerates is aging.

Back now to emphysema and other obstructive lung

diseases. It is doubtful that nucleic-acid therapy will cure these diseases. However, compared with the usual drug therapies, it can be a safer, more effective way of allowing the patient to breathe more easily and guard against dangerous infections. More important, since these diseases afflict the old more than the young, the nucleic acid way of preserving youth can be reasonably expected to help prevent these diseases from beginning.

Once an obstructive disease of the lungs like emphysema or chronic bronchitis sets in, nucleic-acid therapy does two significant things: It permits the body to make more complete use of the oxygen breathed in, and it loosens the cough, thus reducing uncomfortable congestion.

Here is what it did for one patient, a 62-year-old man who was easily winded going up a few stairs, even walking. He had suffered like this for five years before he gave up smoking. Six months later he was no better. The bronchodilators and potassium iodide which he had been taking (the usual treatment for emphysema) were of little use. He had almost forgotten what it was like to breathe normally and feel well. Then he began the nucleic-acid therapy—concentrated RNA plus vitamins.

Two weeks went by before improvement began. He could exercise with less fatigue and less gasping for breath. Six weeks after he began the treatment he could climb two flights of steps with only mild shortness of breath, and he returned to a normal work schedule. His cough was loosened and he felt the relief of less congested lungs. X rays showed this man's lungs damaged by moderately advanced emphysema; nevertheless, after six weeks he was restored to vigor and felt dramatically more comfortable.

Of course, degenerative diseases rarely come alone in old age; little wonder, since they are manifestations of the same underlying condition. However, since they need not be treated one at a time but with a single course of therapy using nutrients natural to the body, treatment is simpler and far safer than conventional drug therapy. A case in point:

A 66-year-old woman, a nonsmoker, had for years suffered from chronic bronchitis, with the coughing and shortness of breath that accompany it. For the past fifteen years her condition had gradually worsened, and for the past four years she gasped for breath even while resting. The usual medications—brochodilators, potassium iodide, and antibiotics—helped some, but not much. X rays showed lung damage typical of her condition.

In addition there was moderate edema of the ankles, a swelling caused by fluid accumulation in the tissues. Edema plus electrocardiograph findings spelled congestive heart failure. Except for the antibiotics, the conventional drugs were stopped and nucleic-acid therapy begun, the same as that used on the 62-year-old emphysema patient. After a week she said she could exercise a little more than before with less shortness of breath. The RNA dosages were increased (from three to four times a week) and she improved still more, enough, in fact, for her to return to normal life with far less coughing, more comfortable breathing, and reduced swelling of the ankles, which had been caused by the congestive heart failure.

What we are dealing with here is a highly significant effect of the nucleic-acid therapy: It permits the body to perform better with less oxygen; or, to say the same thing differently, to make more efficient use of the oxygen we breathe. Let us turn briefly to an experiment with mice to prove this.

What you are about to read is not pretty and causes medical researchers more anguish than many care to talk about. But it is the sort of thing, however ugly it may be, which leads to lifesaving knowledge and must, regrettably, go on.

Fourteen mice were deprived of fresh air. Seven of them had been treated with nucleic acids; for purposes of comparison seven had not been treated. They were sealed in individual glass jars and their survival time recorded.

The experimental mice, those treated with nucleic acids, survived 48 percent longer than the others, and they were much more active through the experiment. One eccentric mouse on nucleic acids was, for reasons of his own, less active than any of his fellows. However, he too lived almost twice as long as the ones who were not treated with nucleic acids.

In another test using twelve mice, the experimental ones survived 45 percent longer, though this time, and in later experiments, I came to recognize the onset of death and released them just in time.

It is interesting (and less disturbing) to note that Charles Darwin more than a century ago reported that Andean Indians traveling to high altitudes, where the air is thin, eat onions as a remedy for altitude sickness. Onions are rich in nucleic acids.

9

New Hope
for Victims of
Heart Disease

Life is uncertain for all of us, but for the heart patient this uncertainty is something he is vividly aware of all the time. No one, not even his doctors, can predict when a fatal attack will strike. One medication after another, diet after diet have been tried, but one fact remains: Heart disease kills more people in the United States than all other causes of death combined.

Why do hearts give out? Cholesterol formation? Some say yes, and some say no, with the weight of evidence favoring the yeses. Age, race, heredity, high blood pressure, cigarette smoking, stress, diet, plus other diseases like diabetes may all, alone or in combination, play a role.

Diets high in unsaturated fats—diets including fish, chicken, and other high-protein, low-fat foods—are useful in reducing the chance of heart attacks. Careful medical studies and statistics show this. Many people are led to believe that these are scientific studies proving the effectiveness of the well-known "low-fat" diets. However, as careful as these studies are, they are not truly scientific. The diets with the most promising results have two things in common: They are low in fats and they have higher-than-normal quantities of nucleic acids. The studies emphasize only what the diets exclude—fats—and ignore what they include—nucleic acids. Had there only been more careful investigation of these diets by teams of investigators with sophisticated clinical facilities available to them, which I do not have, great floodgates of medical knowledge would have been opened.

Let us return to those sixteen patients mentioned in the first chapter, and to the 49-year-old man who was one of them. These patients, you will recall, were on a nucleic-acid-rich diet. The 49-year-old man who could not walk more than half a city block without crippling chest pains had for some time been on medication plus a low-fat diet before he began the nucleic-acid fish diet. His condition was steadily deteriorating, but four weeks after he started the nucleic acid diet, improvement began and continued. Now, as I noted, he walks a mile or more without pain. When he does anything more strenuous and pain does occur, it is milder and does not last as long.

Very simple logic would lead us to conclude that what made the new diet work and the old diet fail was not what they had in common, foods low in saturated fats. We must look for the difference between them— the vastly larger nucleic-acid content of the diet that worked.

Scores of my patients suffering from angina pectoris have had similar results, some from the diet alone, some from nucleic-acid extracts plus other nutrients.

However, angina pectoris is not the only heart disease. Heart failure along with its symptoms—swollen ankles, breathlessness, fatigue—was spectacularly relieved in fifty patients. Their ages ranged from 42 to 97 years, with most in their 60s and 70s. I treated them with the extracts and vitamins which, as I mentioned earlier, operate on the same principle as the diet, but are much stronger and require medical supervision.

What I learned from these patients is that the higher the dosage of nucleic acid, the better the results.

For example, an 83-year-old man had had a heart attack seven years before nucleic-acid therapy began, and for four years he had been suffering from shortness of breath. Simply walking half a city block left him gasping for air. He slept on three or four pillows to make breathing a little easier at night.

A physical examination revealed swollen ankles and feet, lung congestion, plus other symptoms of heart failure. His nucleic-acid treatment started with 1½ grains of RNA daily plus vitamins. In three weeks there was some improvement but not enough. The dosage was raised to 9 grains five days a week, plus an alkalizer to keep acidity down and some magnesium oxide to prevent kidney stones. I gave him no drugs.

Two weeks after the RNA was increased he could walk fifteen city blocks without troubled breathing. His color improved. His lungs were clear of congestion. The swelling disappeared from his ankles and feet. An electrocardiogram two months later showed marked improvement in heart performance. After two-and-a-half months of this treatment, the RNA was stopped for three weeks. The first week he felt no different, but the second and third weeks his shortness of breath began to return and the RNA treatment was resumed. Once again the symptoms disappeared.

In the vast majority of heart patients I have treated with nucleic acids, there was a rapid reduction of blood cholesterol and, more important, a sharp improvement in their overall health.

A WORD OF WARNING: If you are under medical care for a heart condition, do not discontinue your medication simply because you have started this diet. In two to four weeks you will begin to feel better because you will actually be healthier. However, let your doctor confirm this so he can make adjustments in your medication. DO NOT try it yourself.

10

Cholesterol and the No-Aging Diet

Cholesterol is a kind of fat. It has a bad name because of its suspected role in heart disease. Although the findings are not conclusive, they are strong enough to lead any sensible person to avoid foods which might build up high levels of cholesterol in the blood, foods (like bacon) which are high in saturated fats. (Saturated fats are solid animal fats; unsaturated fats are vegetable oils.)

I have found that widely used low-fat diets, while they help, are not good enough. My diet is also low in saturated fats but, more important, it is high in nucleic acids and related biochemicals, which I have found to lower blood cholesterol drastically. In fact, as I mentioned earlier, it may very well be that an important reason why some of these low-fat diets work is that they are a little richer in nucleic acids and related substances than the ordinary diets of most Americans. Interestingly, my work during the past decade has shown that sardines are the most powerful part of the nucleic acid diet in lowering cholesterol.

Why do nucleic acids lower cholesterol? You will remember that the principal work of nucleic acids is to increase the energy in our cells, which leads them to manufacture more ATP. ATP, formed in the electron-transport chain of the cells, is the main supplier and carrier of our bodies' energy. Step up the electron-transport chain and more ATP results.

Two of the key chemicals in this chain contain another chemical from which cholesterol is made—isoprene.

If isoprene is necessary to form parts of the electron-transport chain, which in turn is necessary to the healthy functioning of our bodies, and on the other hand if isoprene makes cholesterol, is this not a self-destruct mechanism in our bodies with which we dare not interfere? No, this would be true only if we cut down production of isoprene. The answer, which I developed in 1973, is really simple and fits neatly into my general theory of aging and degenerative diseases. It is to force isoprene to do one thing and not another—to manufacture the two chemicals necessary to the electron-transport chain and not to make cholesterol.

You will recall that the electron-transport chain gets its energy from the nine-step Krebs cycle. In the first step of this cycle is acetyl coenzyme A. It is this that creates isoprene. Isoprene can be channeled into creating coenzyme Q and the cytochromes, two chemicals necessary to the electron-transport chain; or, if the chain is not efficiently using these chemicals, it can form cholesterol.

For energy to make it operate efficiently, the chain needs plenty of ATP, as we have seen earlier. Nucleic acids lead to increased production of ATP. To produce ATP, the chain needs a full supply of its components so that it can use the isoprene in more productive ways, such as helping build parts of the electron-transport chain, leaving less for cholesterol formation.* This, in

---

* Isoprenes are also basic in the structure of other molecules in the cell. Among these isoprenes are the dolichol phosphates which, working in cooperation with nucleic acids, are important in creating cell membranes. High nucleic-acid intake leads to using isoprenes more for dolichol phosphate production and less for cholesterol formation. In fact, an electron-transport chain made more active by nucleic acids will oxidize more acetyl coenzyme A, leaving less for production of isoprenes; those that are left will be used in greater proportion to make components of the electron-transport chain than in making cholesterol.

grossly simplified terms, is why the no-aging diet is so effective in lowering cholesterol levels in the blood.

My patients with arteriosclerosis are helped in two ways by nucleic acids. These patients suffer from a thickening and hardening of their arteries which can lead to heart damage and brain damage. Some of the more frequent symptoms are loss of memory and an unhealthy looking skin pallor, loss of muscle strength, particularly in the legs, plus the pain of angina pectoris. In most cases they have very high blood cholesterol levels. Nucleic acids lower cholesterol levels. Equally important, the brain, along with the heart and other muscles, is able to make more efficient use of smaller quantities of oxygen. This is important because there is less oxygen-carrying blood flowing through the thickened arteries. You have already read something about this in the chapter "Eat Better; You'll Breathe Easier," which described some of the other benefits of better oxygen use by our bodies as a result of nucleic acids.

11
A New Approach to Diabetes

For every known diabetic in the United States there is probably another who is unaware of having the disease. Altogether, according to an estimate by the Public Health Service, there are about four or more million diabetics in the U.S.

While diabetes is the known cause of scores of life-ruining diseases, the cause of diabetes itself is not known. Simply pointing to inefficient or insufficient insulin production is not enough. We must know what causes *that*. Meanwhile, treatment for diabetes has hardly advanced since insulin was isolated forty years ago.

It is known, for instance, that the diabetic does not metabolize sugar, fat, and protein well, and he must therefore follow rigidly controlled diets and take insulin to improve his metabolism. The symptoms rather than the disease are treated. Meanwhile, the degenerative diseases that result take a melancholy toll. Diabetes is the eighth leading cause of death.

Heart disease, seriously impaired circulation often leading to gangrene, kidney failure, and blindness are a few of the complications of diabetes. It is the third leading cause of blindness.

Because nucleic acids permit the body to utilize oxygen more effectively and help repair damaged tissue, I have used them in keeping the disease at bay—not curing it, but considerably reducing the damage it does.

My treatment involves the standard dietary restrictions and medications plus RNA and vitamins. Eighteen patients 25 to 80 years of age were helped in this way. Those with heart disease were dramatically helped, and the excessive fatigue which characterizes the disease was eliminated. Abnormally occurring pain in the legs of elderly patients during fairly mild exertion, known as intermittent claudication, was relieved or eliminated.

After two to four months, coldness of the legs and feet caused by impaired circulation completely disappeared, and there were fewer infections stemming from the poor circulation.

Three patients suffering from diabetes-caused nerve disorders did not improve in respect to these particular disorders, though one of them was helped by another regime which included heparin, an anticoagulant, crude fiber, B complex, choline, and unflavored gelatin along with the RNA. However, they were all relieved of other symptoms.

More frequently, peripheral nerve damage (numbness) can be treated successfully with the nucleic acid diet, a strong B-complex tablet, plus choline and inositol. The choline and inositol can be taken in 500-mg. tablets one or more times a day. (In research unrelated to my work on nucleic acids, I have found that adding magnesium glycerophosphate to this therapy produces even more striking results. These three substances— choline, inositol, and magnesium glycerophosphate— are required by the body to produce a basic part of nerve structure, the phospholipids.)

One patient, a 25-year-old woman, had outstanding results. Her diabetes had recently been diagnosed. She was taking antisugar tablets and was on the usual restricted diet. Still, her urine was ominously burdened with sugar. With nucleic acid extracts plus the nucleic acid diet and vitamins, her urine became normal after three weeks and remained that way. After six weeks it was possible to advise her to discontinue the tablets.

Diabetes has so many degenerative aspects that it is like many degenerative diseases lumped into one. Here is the way I believe it works:

In degenerative diseases and in aging (which I believe to be very closely related) there is less oxygen-using metabolism and more non-oxygen-using metabolism, largely because of a block in the Krebs cycle or electron transport chain. This means that some NADH (a reduced form of NAD, nicotinamide adenine dinucleotide) and similar molecules are not fully oxidized to form ATP, the high-energy molecule. The oxidation (or burning) of glucose and other cellular materials such as fats produces the hydrogen (the H), which is added on to NAD to form NADH, the reduced nicotinamide adenine dinucleotide.

My investigations have suggested that the NADH produced in the less-oxygen-using metabolism is a critically guilty molecule in producing growth of cancer cells. Also—this is relevant to diabetes—NADH and NADH-like molecules, which play beneficial roles normally, play actively sinister roles for diabetics in the production of sugar complexes known as mucoproteins, which form a membrane inside tiny blood vessels. The thickening of this membrane is the basic lesion of diabetes. The same molecules also stimulate production of cholesterol and fats which, in diabetes, are often found in high concentrations.

This thickening of the blood-vessel membranes interferes with blood circulation, which in turn reduces the cells' oxygen supply—which in turn leads to less ATP production from NADH—a truly vicious cycle. Meanwhile, impaired circulation leads to other complications of diabetes such as blindness, calluses, sensitivity to the cold, and lowered resistance to infections.

You have probably been hearing quite a bit about lecithin lately. Diabetics should know more about it. It is a good source of choline and inositol, two B vitamins which I use in treating diabetes, particularly its nerve disorders. It is also useful in reducing cholesterol. Part of the lecithin molecule is glycerol. With the Krebs cycle blocked, glycerol finds a way around the block and thereby fails to become part of the lecithin molecule, thus reducing normal lecithin production.

Buying lecithin at your drugstore is not the answer to this problem. Most of the lecithin now being advertised is a vegetable product which has fatty acids different from those which our bodies make or use for proper nerve and cell structure. This can make the diabetic's condition worse in some respects, particularly his nerve disorders, because he does not metabolize fats well.

The way I have found to interfere with the vicious cycle mentioned above is to step up the oxygen-using metabolism, thus increasing ATP production. To do this I prescribe nutrients rich in nucleic acids (the diet with or without nucleic acid extracts) plus vitamins, particularly the B complex. For those with peripheral nerve damage I add magnesium glycerophosphate, as I mentioned earlier.

Surely this new approach suggests a direction for major new investigations by research organizations with more extensive facilities than I have.

12

How the No-Aging Diet Can Help Osteoarthritis

Of the various forms of arthritis, osteo is the most frequent. It is a degenerative joint disease. The connective tissues become dry and fibrous and, during flare-ups, there is painful inflammation.

The attack on the disease must be made on two fronts: one to repair damaged connective tissues, and the other to prevent or relieve inflammation.

The joint tissue (collagen) is protein with a chain of various sugar molecules linked to it. Much of the linking is done by enzymes containing manganese. The treatment, therefore, involves nucleic acid to build up the protein and manganese to link up the sugars and help the body create necessary enzymes.

To help the body create the sugars, a number of vitamins are necessary. Biotin is prominent among them. A key vitamin in all this, also, is niacinamide, which we mentioned earlier.

Vitamin C, meanwhile, working with iron, transforms one amino acid (proline) to another (hydroxyproline) which is vital to rebuilding connective tissue.

In other words, nucleic acid, vitamins (particularly biotin and C), plus trace minerals are the first line of attack.

The second line of attack, this one against inflammation, also depends on a complex web of interactions leading up to coenzyme A. This coenzyme contains pantothenic acid, a B vitamin which the body uses to produce hormones needed to reduce inflammation. Other steps along the way may depend on vitamin C.

Now for the key question: How can we use all this bewildering information?

If you have a family history of osteoarthritis and do not have it yet, or if you already have a very mild case, the following, in addition to the diet, will help:

Take a teaspoonful of brewer's yeast (or six to ten tablets) per day. It contains nucleic acids and B vitamins.

Take one tablespoon of blackstrap molasses per day. This is rich in vitamins and minerals as well as sugar.

Take one tablespoon of natural wheat germ per day. This too is rich in trace minerals as well as vitamins.

Instead of sugar in coffee and tea, use honey, which contains manganese.

Where the no-aging diet calls for fruit juices, avoid orange, grapefruit, lime, or lemon juice. These, for reasons not yet understood, seem to cause osteoarthritis to flare up.

In addition to the multivitamin tablet, take 250 mg. a day of pantothenic acid and 500 mg. of vitamin C.

One other helpful food is mushrooms. These contain copper, which is important for building up proper joint proteins.

If you have a serious case of arthritis, the above regime will probably not be of any significant help. You will need more pantothenic acid, and prolonged higher dosages can be harmful to you unless you are under a doctor's care. Besides, since vitamins do not work alone but in conjunction with each other, too much of one vitamin can deplete the others. They must be in balance. You will need a physician to advise you on this balance.

13

A No-Aging Diet for Vegetarians

It used to be said that those who chose vegetarianism as a way of life did so simply because it seemed to them uncivilized to kill animals. This is what Thoreau had in mind when he wrote in *Walden*:

> I have no doubt that it is a part of the destiny of the human race, in its gradual improvement, to leave off eating animals, as surely as the savage tribes have left off eating each other when they came in contact with the more civilized.

This is still a widespread, in fact growing, reason for vegetarianism. But there is now another, and in my opinion more compelling, one—meat is an expensive, inefficient nutrient for a growing world population. If we all became vegetarians, food would be cheaper and vastly more abundant. We cannot ignore the fact that about ten times the food value we get from meat has been used to produce it.

From a medical point of view, there is a lot to be said for vegetarian diets. They are low in fat and cholesterol, and they can be perfectly well balanced. The trick to balancing them is to include the necessary amino acids which the body needs to make proteins.

Of all the amino acids—there are twenty important ones—our adult bodies can produce twelve. The remaining eight must come from outside the body. They are called "essential" amino acids because they are necessary parts of a healthy diet. Illness results from the lack of any one of them.

Meat and fish contain all eight; few vegetables do. This is where vegetarians can go tragically wrong. No one vegetable is enough. No one type of vegetable is enough. The vegetarian needs a proper balance of them at each meal. A combination of grains and beans, for instance, supplies all the essential amino acids provided they are taken at the same time. A breakfast of cereals and a lunch of beans will not work. Cereal with milk for breakfast, lentil soup with bread for lunch is the way to do it.

Here is the basic nutritional rule for vegetarians to live by: Each meal must include at least one of the following three combinations:

1. grains with milk products
2. legumes (e.g. beans, peas, lentils) with grains
3. nuts and seeds with legumes

Where one part of these combinations is weak in amino acids, the other part is strong. For a more detailed discussion of the amino-acid content of foods, I recommend a highly readable book by Frances Moore Lappé, *Diet for a Small Planet* (Ballantine Books). It contains a wide range of meatless recipes, each employing at least one of the above combinations.

There is one other pitfall in the vegetarian diet: a shortage of B vitamins, particularly B_{12}. This is easy to avoid with a therapeutic-strength multivitamin capsule—an absolute must.

Where do vegetables like lettuce and carrots come in? And fruits? They are low in amino acids, but high in vitamins and minerals—some, as you will see, in nucleic acids.

If you are willing to eat fish, things are simple for you. Follow the diet in Chapter Four with only one change: eliminate liver once a week. In its place, eat some cod or halibut or salmon.

If you are a strict vegetarian and eat neither meat nor fish, here is a diet that will provide the necessary nucleic acids:

1. Have one meal with a liberal portion of asparagus three times a week,

2. another meal with a generous portion of mushrooms three times a week,

3. and, also three times a week, a meal with beets, beet juice, or borscht.

4. Have collard greens, cauliflower, spinach, soybean sprouts, or turnip greens as part of your main meal four times a week.

Every day have

5. a glass of fruit or vegetable juice,

6. two glasses of milk, preferably skimmed,

7. at least four glasses of water,

8. one therapeutic-strength multivitamin capsule with the main meal,

9. and finally, don't forget to include, for each meal, one of the three combinations mentioned earlier.

One more word of special advice to strict vegetarians: You have a special need to learn all you can about nutrition because there are dangers in eating only vegetables, as I have already pointed out. You can overcome these dangers and eat ethically and healthfully (and interestingly), but you should learn much more about nutrition than I have written here. My attention is necessarily focused sharply on nucleic acids; there is obviously more to nutrition than that.

14

Make Up Your Own No-Aging Diet

To achieve the most youthful, healthy appearance, along with good health itself, we need one to one and a half grams of nucleic acid per day. It does not matter much whether they come from sardines or soybeans, provided we avoid excessive cholesterol and calories. I say it does not matter much; it does matter some. Sardines, for example, are richer in minerals than soybeans and my experience shows that they have a remarkable ability to lower cholesterol. Besides, they are lower on the food chain than bigger fish like tuna, and are therefore less likely to contain man-made pollutants like insecticides. Here is why: Big fish eat smaller fish, smaller fish eat still smaller fish, each with some pollutants stored in its body. The smaller the fish, the closer it is to the bottom of the food chain where there are less pollutants to eat.

However, many people cannot stomach sardines or liver, or some of the other foods I have recommended. If you are one of them, the table which follows will help you choose other foods adding up to one or one and a half grams, as in a Chinese menu, from the same column.

About the table: Until the very eleventh hour of this book's publication I knew of no table listing the nucleic acid content of foods. As far as I knew, dietary nucleic acids had been entirely ignored by nutritionists and medical researchers other than in special instances, as in gout.

I therefore had to derive a table of my own from other tables of the purine content of foods. When purines are present, so are nucleic acids. When you multiply the purine content of foods by 3.5, you get the approximate nucleic acid content.

It is important for physicians to know about purines because they often advise their patients with gout to avoid them. However, even data on purine content is hard to come by.

In the November 1939 issue of the *Journal of the American Dietetic Association,* a low-purine diet was published with the following comment:

> A review of the available literature regarding the purine . . . content of foods revealed a distressing paucity of usable figures and consistent values. . . . In an attempt to obtain the most recent figures available, we solicited aid from many outstanding authorities throughout the United States. We found that none were using . . . purine calculations, or could add to the common list of references, or would attempt to evaluate comparatively the tables given in current texts.

This was in 1939. Thirty years later, Dorothea Turner wrote in the fourth edition of *Handbook of Diet Therapy* (published by the University of Chicago Press for the American Dietetic Association):

> A review of the available literature regarding the purine content . . . of foods revealed a distressing paucity of usable figures and consistent values. . . .
>
> In an attempt to obtain the most recent figures available, aid was solicited from outstanding authorities throughout the United States. It was found that none were using purine calculations or could add to the common list of references, or would attempt to evaluate comparatively the tables given in current texts.

Thirty years of progress!

However, while I was reading the printer's proofs of this book, Dr. Hendler, who wrote the foreword, providentially led me to Dr. A. J. Clifford, Professor of Nutrition at the University of California at Davis. Dr. Clifford had very recently made a detailed study of the chemistry of various foods, including their RNA content. He generously permitted me to list his findings in the following table.

I derived the RNA content of some foods not included in Dr. Clifford's study from purine tables.

The following foods, not included in Dr. Clifford's study, are also rich in nucleic acids as indicated by their purine content:

most fish	wheat germ
meat extracts	bran
nuts	asparagus
poultry (dark meat)	mushrooms
spinach	radishes
oatmeal	onions

On the other hand, foods low in nucleic acids, although in many cases rich in other important nutrients, are:

most vegetables	cheese*
fruits	natural cereals
eggs*	butter*
milk	other fats

Although beets, like most vegetables, are not high in nucleic acids they are an important part of my diet. They contain an amino acid which the body uses to create its own nucleic acid, plus another nutrient important to brain function.

One facet of Dr. Clifford's findings struck my eye

* Fairly high in cholesterol.

NUCLEIC ACID
CONTENT OF FOODS

FOODS	RNA	FOODS	RNA
ORGAN MEATS			
chicken liver	402*	lamb liver	88*
beef liver	268*	beef brain	61*
pork liver	259*	lamb heart	50
chicken heart	187	beef heart	49
beef kidney	134*		
FRESH SEAFOODS			
sardines	343	mackerel	203
anchovies	341	squid	100*
salmon	289	clams	85*
CANNED SEAFOODS			
sardines	590	salmon	26
oysters	239*	shrimp	10*
mackerel	122	anchovies	6
herring	82	tuna	5
clams	44*		
DRIED LEGUMES			
pinto beans	485	great northern	
lentils	484	beans	284
garbanzo beans	356	cranberry beans	248
blackeye peas	306	baby lima beans	190
small white		split peas	173
beans	305	red beans	140
large lima			
beans	293		

* Fairly high in cholesterol, but rich in important nutrients.

immediately: the dramatically sharp drop in RNA content of canned versus fresh seafoods. Fresh anchovies, clams, mackerel, and salmon are all vastly richer in RNA than when they are canned, but this is not true with sardines. Unaccountably, canned sardines have more RNA than fresh ones.

Sardines stand out in another significant respect: Dr. Clifford found that they contain a very high level of xanthine, a derivative of RNA, and that when he gave xanthine to volunteers they showed little rise in uric acid levels. Until his important study, the opposite would have been expected.

My own experience with sardines has been that they—more than any other food—lower cholesterol and quickly provide patients with greater energy.

I believe there is a significant connection between Dr. Clifford's findings and mine. His provide me with the basis for theorizing that xanthine, instead of creating uric acid like other RNA constituents, creates guanosine diphosphate, which is critical to the working of the Krebs cycle. When this cycle is operating at peak efficiency, you will recall, it can reverse or slow down the aging process and combat degenerative diseases.

In short, there is growing scientific evidence of the special importance of sardines in our diet. Unlike medicines that are often used to control degenerative diseases, sardines show no hazardous side effects.

15
Some Other
Theories
of
Aging

A number of theories of aging, and some therapies, have gained a fair measure of renown lately. A question you might ask is, "How does the theory presented in this book—that loss of energy in the cell is the basic cause of aging and degenerative diseases—square with them?"

Let's take the most prominent theory first. You may have heard about it in relation to vitamin E. Aging, according to this theory, is caused by free radicals and oxidative processes.

A free radical is a wildly active molecule with a missing electron. It lives a career of restless destruction by reacting promiscuously with other molecules, causing them to become free radicals too. Free radicals enter our bodies mainly from foods which have been oxidized (by, for example, X rays, cosmic rays, and nuclear fallout). Once in the body, they damage DNA as well as other cell structures.

Since DNA is the cell's blueprint for building new cells, once it is damaged it designs other damaged cells which, in turn, design other damaged ones. Vitamin E, an antioxidant, tends to deactivate free radicals and thus reduce the rate of damage. Other antioxidants are vitamin C and the trace element selenium.

My opinion is that the free-radical theory represents a part of the truth. Cells are damaged by more than free radicals. Stress, viruses, poor nutrition, are other causes.

As for the antioxidant therapy, there is some evidence that it may slow down the rate of cell damage. My nutritional therapy, which includes vitamins in abundance, not only slows down the rate of damage, but it repairs the damage once it occurs. It does this in three ways: first by providing the cell with energy for self-repair; second by providing the materials for building up coenzymes; and third by providing ready-made structural units for the body's own nucleic acids.

Another closely related theory, one which also calls for the use of vitamin E, is the oxidation theory. When paper turns brown and brittle, when rubber loses its snap, when iron rusts and copper turns green, when anything burns, oxidation has done it. Whenever oxygen joins a molecule, the process is known as oxidation. This changes the molecule, makes it behave differently. If the molecule is part of our body, it becomes less efficient or actually harmful when oxidized. This, according to the oxidation theory, is the root cause of aging. Vitamin E slows down oxidation, hence retards aging. Once again, I see this theory as part of the truth and not inconsistent with mine. However, again, the therapy stemming from it does not, as mine does, repair damage already done.

A particularly interesting theory holds that protein molecules, which are long chains of amino acids, become linked with other protein molecules. The doubled or tripled molecules that result are unnatural to the body. They gum up the cell with useless, endangering debris. Work on preventing this linking, and other work on disconnecting the links, is now underway by several research groups, and the results so far appear promising. Once again, this theory of cellular damage is not inconsistent with mine, though research into ways of repairing the damage appears to be taking a totally different tack.

You have probably heard of the work of Dr. Anna Aslan, a Rumanian physician. She reported important antiaging results from injections of procaines along with B vitamins. The critical reason for the effectiveness of this therapy, I believe, is that through a complex series of chemical reactions, five of the nine basic units of the purine molecule may be created. Purine, you will recall, plays a key role in creating nucleic acids and many important coenzymes.

You may also have heard of work done in the Soviet Union with vitamin B_{15} (pangamic acid). Large daily injections of this vitamin are reported to be useful in treating several degenerative diseases, including hardening of the arteries. Pangamic acid contains methyl groups which, along with folic acid, help create purines which contain nucleic acids. Both B_{15} and procaine owe much of their effectiveness to their ability to put into motion bodily processes which create nucleic acids.

A more recent theory of aging appears related to some promising research of my own. The theory concerns the outer surface, the membrane of the cell. On this surface are receptors, things which respond to stimuli from hormones produced by several of the body's glands.

What these receptors are and what they look like is less understood than what they do. We can think of them as doing for the cell pretty much what an antenna does for a radio. They are probably made of the same materials as the membrane itself, though in different proportions—phospholipids, proteins, and sugar complexes.

The basic structure of these phospholipids is derived mostly from glycerol phosphate. However, I believe that when a damaged cell needs extra energy, as it often does, the glycerol phosphate provides this energy (by being oxidized in the cell and becoming ATP) and less of it is available for properly making the lipids. This leads to a build-up of damage not only to the receptors but to the membrane, both inside and out.

The outer membrane is more than just a packaging for the cell. Like the interior membranes, it is a highly active part of the cell, containing enzymes basic to all aspects of the body's metabolism.

My basic hypothesis is that glycerol phosphate from

outside the body may repair damaged cell membranes, including the receptors. To test this I began a series of very promising experiments: I swallowed fairly high doses of glycerol phosphate. The results were similar in some respects to nucleic acid therapy! My skin became even tighter and younger looking and my near vision, which often deteriorates with age, improved sharply.

Other similar experiments are providing me with strong indications that the nervous system and other organs are also strongly improved this way.

Glycerol phosphate is not itself a nutrient but is made from nutrients by our cells. Therefore, before routinely incorporating this into any therapy, much more work is necessary to better understand what takes place when the substance is administered. What I hope for is that a course of treatment separate from nucleic acid therapy will result and that the two together may prove to be more than twice as effective as either one alone.

All of these theories are essentially mechanistic—they deal with the action of one physical substance on another. A vastly different approach to aging and disease, one which fascinates me but about which I know little, is the effect of the mind on the body. My emphasis is on the body side of this interaction. However, I believe the current explosion of interest in exploring the healing powers of the mind is demonstrating a hitherto unsuspected power of the mind side of this interaction. I am thinking of mind control, transcendental meditation, and biofeedback among others. One day I expect that this approach will profoundly affect the practice of "medicine."

Another development, centuries old, is acupuncture. The Western medical world has only recently made grudging admission of its usefulness, especially for pain. New ideas often require more than proof to become accepted; they require a kind of social respectability which is stubbornly difficult to come by.

16

Toward
a
Healthier
Future

More people are living longer—thanks to advances in medicine; and more people than ever before are in poor health. This is not too surprising when we consider that diseases select older victims more than younger ones and there are more older ones around now.

When we find whatever it is that makes old bodies more hospitable to diseases than young ones, we will have a single line of attack against these diseases. Today we do little more than attack the symptoms, often at terrible cost to the patient's health.

The diet is not the final answer, nor are the more powerful nucleic acid extracts. But clearly they suggest where to look for that single line of attack. It lies in the neglected area of nutrition, of nourishing the body so that its cells will have the energy to repair themselves.

You might wonder why, with the dramatic results you have just read about, a vast scientific effort—even on the scale of the famed Manhattan Project—has not been launched to investigate them. Cynical answers about the venality or ignorance of the medical profession do not wash. Physicians sincerely want to cure their patients and medical researchers really want to achieve breakthroughs.

Why, then, have the efforts of the professional lifetime of one physician failed to attract the attention of his colleagues? Why has the medical profession ignored them?

There are several reasons. One is that medical doctors study medicine, not nutrition. Another, perhaps more important, is that they have spent lifetimes acquiring useful, in many cases lifesaving, knowledge organized around theories with which this nutritional approach is often incompatible. Imagine convincing a busy surgeon to put down his scalpel and learn to treat his patients with nucleic acids.

But what of the pharmaceutical companies? It is unreasonable to look to them. They must make money by making pharmaceuticals. Nature makes nucleic acids.

And the great research organizations? Of course we cannot expect them to accept what to them must appear to be the extravagant claims of a single physician reporting on the experience gained in his own modest practice. But following up on such findings as the ones you have read about here is their job. They have not done it. There is no excuse.

There have been many more spectacular findings than those described in this book which is necessarily limited to those you can profit from through a simple diet. For example: Years ago I gave very high doses of RNA extract to patients at the onset of colds; the colds were knocked out in six to eight hours. I have repeated this experiment many times. It has tremendous implications. It suggests that nucleic acids are effective against viruses. This finding alone warrants more serious research.

Another example: A patient with a rare eye disease, retinitis pigmentosa, was much helped in six weeks with a combination of RNA extracts and the diet. The disease can cause blindness and there is no reliable treatment for it. Of course, this is only one patient, but since the therapy is safe why not try it on others? Three other patients with a common form of glaucoma were improved enough to discontinue eye medication.

Major research efforts will begin one day on nucleic-acid therapy, and when this happens medical science will probably be headed in basically different, more promising directions. You will profit in spectacular ways. It is entirely reasonable for you to expect to live

120, perhaps 150 years in good health when this nutritional approach is further improved and becomes the accepted way of maintaining health and repairing it when it is damaged.

Meanwhile, there is no need for you to wait for this medical revolution to come about. The diet is perfectly safe and has been proved effective in slowing down the aging process and returning many who were seriously sick to good health. Maybe we will not reach 150, but at least middle age need no longer be that time of life when we think we will feel better next week.

17

Recipes for the No-Aging Diet

To look better, feel better, and be better are probably your reasons for giving the no-aging diet a try. But if this makes life suddenly turn gray because you do not like some of the foods I have recommended, the diet becomes less of a blessing for you than I want it to be. To avoid this, I am providing a variety of recipes, many of which have been given to me by my patients. You will find many of them unusual and all of them, I hope, interesting enough to try.

SOME SARDINE RECIPES

Let us start with sardines. For some reason these seem to be a masculine food; it is mostly women I have heard say they do not like them. Few, however, continue to dislike sardines after exploring the many ways of serving them.

To begin, we must open the sardine can. I hope you will forgive me if I discuss this briefly, because it is important to those who are on weight-reducing diets. The oil in which the sardines are packed is itself packed with calories. It must be drained off.

Open the can about a quarter of the way, then lean it against something, a saucer perhaps, in the sink with the partially open end down. Do something else for a few minutes while they drain.

If you want to be particularly careful and get rid of still more oil, empty the sardines onto a paper towel and put another paper towel on top.

Now for ways of serving them:

The two most usual ways, I think, are in sandwiches and hors d'oeuvres.

Sardine Sandwich

Two slices of onion rye bread, a slice of sweet onion, the sardines; and you have a sandwich which, with a glass of fruit or vegetable juice or skimmed milk, makes a superbly nourishing lunch.

Hors d'Oeuvre or Canapé

For nutritional reasons, I prefer *hors d'oeuvres variés* to canapés.

The *hors d'oeuvres variés* that I have in mind consist of a plate of varied cold things served before a meal. Nonpurists may make an entire meal of them. Here are some of the things you can use to make up a nourishing and tasty plate:

> sardines
> 1 or 2 tbsp. cooked lentils
> some slightly cooked string beans
> a few beet slices
> cauliflower
> a slice or two of tomato
> a stalk of celery
> a few stalks of asparagus

Over all this sprinkle about a tablespoonful of lemon juice. (Avoid vinegar, which people most frequently use here. It is too acidic for those on a nucleic-acid-rich diet.) If you wish, sprinkle about a teaspoonful of olive oil over everything but the fish.

A Canapé

Mince 5 sweet gherkins and a medium-sized onion. Put them in a bowl and add 5 tbsp. lemon juice.

Add a 3½-oz. can of sardines and an 8-oz. packet of cream cheese.

Blend all this with a fork and use it as a spread on crackers.

Another Canapé

Very lightly toast two slices of white bread and cut each slice into four pieces.

Mash 3½ oz. of sardines with a fork and spread over the bread pieces.

Top with a few small pieces of Swiss cheese.

Bake in a moderate oven (about 350° F) until the cheese melts.

Sardine Hero

Here is a meal-in-itself sandwich with plenty of nourishment:

Cut off a 6- or 7-inch length of French or Italian bread. Slice it lengthwise.

Spread one side with mayonnaise, the other with mustard.

Cover one side with lettuce, tomato slices, and some raw sweet-onion rings and a thin slice of Swiss cheese.

Arrange 3½ oz. of sardines on top of all this, and cover with the other piece of bread.

Sardine Pizza

Almost everyone likes pizza but most people regard it as "junk" food. The truth is it is highly nutritious and not too difficult to make. Here is a way to do it with English muffins:

Ingredients:

2 English muffins
about ½ C. spaghetti sauce
2 tbsp. grated Parmesan and/or Romano cheese
3½-oz. can sardines
garlic powder (optional)
oregano (optional)

Split and toast the English muffins. Cover the muffin pieces with spaghetti sauce, then sprinkle these with a tbsp. of grated cheese.

Break sardines into large pieces and distribute these on the muffin halves.

Cover with more spaghetti sauce and sprinkle again with the remaining cheese. If you wish, add to each a dash of garlic powder and oregano.

Place under broiler (about 3 inches from the flame) until the cheese melts and the sauce bubbles.

Peppers Stuffed with Sardines

Ingredients:

2 large green peppers
3½-oz. can sardines, chopped
1 C. cooked rice
½ medium-sized onion, minced
½ C. tomato sauce
1 egg
salt
pepper

With a paring knife cut a circle around the stem of each of the peppers. Pull out the stems and with a fork or teaspoon scrape away as many of the seeds from the hollow inside as you can. Rinse them out with cold water.

Mix the sardines with the rice, the onion, and the tomato sauce. Beat the egg and add this along with about ½ tsp. of salt and a dash of pepper.

Put this mixture into the hollow peppers, and bake for about 20 minutes at 350°F.

Sardines and Rice

Ingredients:

1 medium onion, sliced
1 green pepper, sliced
3 cloves garlic, minced
3 tbsp. olive oil
3 tbsp. tomato paste
½ C. natural or brown rice
2½ C. boiling water
1 small can carrots and peas
2 3½-oz. cans sardines

Sauté the onion, pepper, and garlic in the olive oil until the pepper and onion become soft.

Add the tomato paste and the rice.

Pour in the water and cook covered over low heat until the water is absorbed.

Add the carrots and peas and sardines. Return to low heat until it becomes hot, then stir it up. Serve with a tossed salad.

Sardines with Gouda Cheese

This makes a superb easy-to-cook main dish for two.

Ingredients:

2 3½-oz. cans sardines
1 lb. spinach
1½ C. skimmed milk
3 tbsp. corn oil margarine
3 tbsp. flour
2 tsp. Worcestershire sauce
¾ C. crumbled Gouda cheese

Drain the sardines into a large frying pan and set the sardines aside.

Wash the spinach and tear it into bite-sized pieces. Heat the sardine oil and pile the spinach onto it. Cover and cook over low heat for five minutes.

While the spinach is cooking put 1 C. of the skimmed milk into a saucepan with the margarine. Heat over very low heat until the margarine melts.

Mix the flour into the rest of the skimmed milk, and pour the mixture slowly into the heating milk while stirring. Add the Worcestershire sauce, and all but 3 tbsp. of the cheese. Continue stirring until cheese melts, making sure the mixture does not boil.

Put the cooked spinach into a greased baking dish, then the sardines on top of the spinach and the cheese sauce on top of everything. Sprinkle the rest of the cheese on this, and bake at 400°F until the cheese melts (about 10 minutes).

Sardine Empanadas

Ingredients:

10 circles of dough (see below)
1 tomato
1 medium-sized onion
1 egg, hard-boiled
3½ oz. sardines
1 tsp. grated Romano and/or Parmesan cheese
oregano
pepper
1 egg, beaten
vegetable oil

You will need 10 circles of dough about ⅛-inch thick and about 5 inches across. There are three ways of providing yourself with the dough. The easiest way is to go to Chinatown and buy sheets of dough for won-ton.

The next easiest (and best) way is to buy uncooked biscuits, which grocery stores sell in cardboard tubes. Powder a chopping board with flour and roll these out. If, like most modern kitchens, yours is without a rolling pin, use a soda bottle.

The hardest way is to make the dough. Mix 2 C. flour with ½ C. meat broth, 1 tsp. salt, and 3 tbsp. margarine. Knead this well, pinch off lumps about half the size of a golf ball, and roll them out.

For the filling, peel the tomato and chop it coarsely, finely chop the onion, coarsely chop the hard-boiled egg, and add the sardines, the grated cheese, a small pinch of oregano, and pepper. Mix it up thoroughly with a fork.

Put about 1½ tbsp. of the filling in the center of each of the dough circles and then fold them over, using the beaten egg to seal the edges.

Put all the empanadas in a preheated oven at 375°F

for five minutes, then brush them with the vegetable oil and continue baking until browned, which should take another 15 minutes.

Two people can consume all this in far less time than it takes to make them.

Sardine Spaghetti Sauce

If you have tried these recipes and are still not convinced that there are many tasty things to do with sardines, you will have to face the fact that you just do not like them. However, there is one more thing to try. It is very simple and hides the flavor of sardines pretty well.

When you make spaghetti with marinara sauce, add 3½ ounces of mashed sardines to the sauce for each serving.

If you use canned marinara sauce, doctor it up with a little Tabasco sauce and a pinch of oregano, and perhaps some garlic.

Of course, you will not want to eat spaghetti as often as you should eat sardines on this diet. That would add up to too many calories. But using this recipe once in a while will help if you find eating sardines unpleasant.

If you like the sardine recipes with cheese, I share your feelings but suggest you not eat more than two of them a week. Most cheeses, particularly the hard ones like Cheddar, Parmesan and Romano, are very high in fats. Other cheeses, like Gouda, though less flavorful, are much lower in fats and safer to eat.

Persons with heart disease, of course, should check with their physicians before including high-fat cheeses in their diets.

You may wonder why all these recipes call for canned sardines. Generally, the more nourishing a food is the more careful we must be about storing it. Fresh sardines, unless you live on the seacoast near where they are caught, are almost unobtainable because they are so difficult to keep from spoiling during shipping.

The no-aging diet calls for small sardines, like the ones from Portugal, not the larger ones that come in oval cans. The smaller ones are richer in nucleic acids. Most of these small sardines come packed in oil. Some are canned in water and are difficult to find but worth looking for. They are less fattening. You can use them in the same recipes as the others. (In Sardines with Gouda Cheese, use vegetable oil for the spinach.)

Some sardines are packed in mustard. These are good, in fact great, but they belong in sandwiches and hors d'oeuvres, not in other recipes.

I have nothing against the larger "sardines" (they are really herring) that come in oval cans; they are simply not quite as rich in nucleic acids as the smaller ones.

SOME FISH RECIPES

How to Cook Fish

By now it comes as no surprise to you that I take fish very seriously. Fish provides many more nutritional advantages than can be discussed here. Fish is packed with vitamins, richer in minerals than meat, easier to digest, provides all the essential amino acids, and is free of fats.

Besides—and this is important since eating should be an interesting experience—fish can be delicious when it is cooked properly.

Two rules to observe: First, be sure the fish is fresh. You can tell by smell and by the fish's eyes. An ammonia odor means the fish is spoiled. Sunken, glazed eyes mean the same thing. The second rule is not to overcook it. Overcooked fish, though it will not lose nucleic acids, will lose some of its vitamin content and flavor.

Hints on Chinese Cooking

Like acupuncture, Chinese cooking has been around for a long time but has only recently been discovered in America. We have many excellent Chinese restaurants, but to the average American the ways of cooking Chinese food remain an inscrutable mystery.

It is really simple. The most difficult part is the shopping; you have to do this in a fairly large city where there is a Chinese market. If you live far from a Chinatown, get to know the owner of a nearby Chinese restaurant. He may be pleased to supply you with the few things you will need.

For the following recipe, you need only three Chinese ingredients: a bag or can of black beans (these are fermented soybeans), a bottle of sesame oil (you will use so little of it the bottle will last for months), and soy sauce (Japanese soy sauce is widely available, far better than the domestic).

Steamed Fish, Chinese Style

One of the more complicated-looking, yet one of the easiest dishes to prepare is steamed fish in black-bean sauce, which is on the menu of many non-chop-suey-type Chinese restaurants. Once you get the hang of it you will be able to sit down to a delicious dinner only half an hour after you come home from the fish market.

Here are the mechanics of steaming a fish:

You need a heat-proof dish about two inches deep and big enough to hold the fish. The fish goes into the dish, the dish goes into a large roasting pan with a cover. Enough water to come up to within about an inch of the top of the dish should be in the roasting pan.

When the water boils, the dish will rattle. To avoid

this, put it on a low rack in the pan, or on two all-metal kitchen knives.

Now for the ingredients:

> 1 medium-sized sea bass
> fresh ginger root
> 3 tbsp. soy sauce
> 3 tbsp. dry sherry
> 1 tsp. sesame oil
> 3 tbsp. peanut oil
> 2 tbsp. Chinese black beans
> 2 or 3 cloves garlic, mashed
> whites of 3 scallions

Put the cleaned, scaled sea bass in the dish. If you wish, the head and tail may be cut off.

Strew about eight nickel-thin slices of ginger around the fish.

Over the fish pour the soy sauce, sherry, sesame oil, and the peanut oil. Lightly rinse the black beans and add these, spreading them around but not on the fish. Add the garlic and the scallions.

Put the dish in the pan. Cover the pan tightly and put it over a high flame. Begin your timing as soon as you hear the water boil. Allow fifteen minutes for the first pound, five minutes per additional pound.

One more word about the mechanics of this: Be careful when you remove the fish. As you take the cover off the roasting pan, hold your head well back to avoid the upward rush of steam.

Lifting the dish from the boiling water can endanger your fingertips. Pour some ice water into the hot water and then use two potholders to quickly lift the dish.

Serve the fish by scooping out large chunks with a tablespoon. When you have finished the top side, simply lift up the tail (or the end where the tail was) and the entire skeleton should come with it, leaving the underside ready to serve.

You will enjoy the nutritious sauce over rice, which is

an almost necessary accompaniment. You may also wish to serve Spinach in Anchovy Sauce (see page 116) and applesauce.

A Cassoulet with Salmon

A cassoulet, as the French make it, is a hearty dish for winter days and big appetites. It is memorably tasty but is not for us. It contains salt pork, pork rind, sausage, lamb, and duck—ingredients which add up to an unacceptably high concentration of saturated fats.

Here is one which takes far less time to make, is far less expensive, and is much more nutritious and almost as tasty—in fact many may prefer it. You can keep it in the refrigerator for a few days, so here's a recipe for five or six servings:

Ingredients:

1 lb. fresh, baby lima beans
2 C. water
1 lb. fresh salmon
1 lb. macaroni
1 green pepper
2 cloves garlic
1 medium-sized onion
4 tbsp. corn oil margarine
2 tbsp. flour
½ C. grated Romano and/or Parmesan cheese

Boil the lima beans, shelled, in lightly salted water to cover for about twenty minutes.

Simmer the salmon in 2 C. water until you can flake it with a fork.

Meanwhile, boil the macaroni according to directions on the package.

Finely chop the pepper, garlic, and onion, and fry them in half of the margarine until they become tender.

Mix the flour into the fluid the salmon was simmered in, and add this to the pepper mixture. Stir until it thickens.

Add the grated cheese and stir until it melts.

Now, grease a casserole with the rest of the margarine and add, in successive layers (make 2 or 3 layers) the macaroni, lima beans, salmon, and sauce. Cover the casserole and bake for about 30 minutes at 350°F.

You can vary this in four ways:

Instead of fresh salmon, use a pound of canned salmon. Add about 1½ C. water to make up the difference in fluid.

Instead of the fluid in which the salmon was boiled, use two cups of skimmed milk.

Instead of fresh lima beans, use canned or frozen beans, preparing according to package directions.

Instead of lima beans, use dried white pea beans. Soak a cup of them in cold water for six hours, then boil them in fresh salted water until they are tender. Depending on the beans, this can take as long as 3 hours.

Finally, add a tablespoon of tomato paste to any of these variations.

Salmon Chowder

Ingredients:

1 green pepper
1 small onion
1 clove garlic
3 tbsp. corn oil margarine
1 8-oz. can of salmon
¾ C. chicken broth
1 bay leaf
thyme
white pepper
3 medium-sized ripe tomatoes

Finely chop the green pepper, onion, and garlic, and fry these in the margarine until they begin to become tender. Drain the fluid from the salmon can into a saucepan, setting the salmon aside. Add the chicken broth, bay leaf, pinch of thyme, and a dash of white pepper. Skin and chop the tomatoes into bite-sized chunks and add. Simmer these ingredients for five minutes.

Meanwhile, break the salmon into large chunks. When the soup has simmered for the five minutes, add the salmon and simmer for 15 minutes more.

This will make 2 to 3 good-sized servings.

Two Mixed-Seafood Soups

We come now to two of the most spectacular ways of preparing seafood, both of them main courses.

The first comes from the Mediterranean, where each seaport has its own way of preparing a soup from the bounty of its waters. Marseilles has its bouillabaisse, which is the most famous of all; yet there are almost as many ways of preparing bouillabaisse as there are persons who cook it. You, too, can vary the recipe to suit your taste and the availability of ingredients.

If you are like most Americans, the idea of eating squid is repellent. Leave it out of the recipe if you must, but allow me to make a brief plea for it.

Of all forms of life on earth, pound for pound nature produces more squid than anything else. The smaller varieties, the ones we eat, are low on the food chain. They are rich in nucleic acids and—a fact unknown to most Americans—they have a flavor delicately reminiscent of the sea. You can buy them at most fish markets which serve a Chinese, Latin-American, or Mediterranean clientele. If you can, buy them already cleaned and cut up.

If you must clean them yourself, remove the tentacles and cut them into inch-long pieces. Cut off the area around the eye and discard it. What you have remaining is a tube. Turn it inside out and scrape away the gelatinous material and the strip of cartilage. Then cut the tube into rings about a half inch wide.

Mixed Seafood Soup, Mediterranean Style

This recipe will serve about six persons.

Ingredients:

4 tbsp. corn oil margarine
4 cloves garlic, crushed
1 or 2 dried chili peppers
2 C. clam broth
2 lobster tails, split or quartered
1 lb. squid
1 dozen small clams
½ lb. shrimp
fillets of 1 small sea bass
2 tbsp. parsley
4 heaping tbsp. unflavored bread crumbs

In a big saucepan melt the margarine and add the garlic and chili peppers.

About two minutes later add the clam broth. When the clam broth boils, add the lobster tails.

Three minutes later add squid and clams. As soon as this boils, add the shrimp and the sea bass fillets cut into bite-sized pieces.

Two minutes after this comes to a boil add the chopped parsley and bread crumbs. Stir well for a minute and serve.

The number of substitutions you can make are almost endless. Eliminate any one thing and you still have a superb soup. Eliminate any two things and you have a good soup. Or use mussels instead of clams, fillet of sole or cod or halibut instead of sea bass, scallops instead of shrimp, chicken broth instead of clam broth (which is done in Bilbao).

Mixed Seafood Soup, Chinese Style

Here are the only changes you need to make to convert Mixed Seafood Soup, Mediterranean Style, to a fascinating Chinese main dish:

In the beginning use peanut oil instead of margarine, and add 2 tbsp. finely chopped fresh ginger; then add only 1 C. clam broth.

Eliminate the bread crumbs.

At the very end, when you add the parsley, pour in one more cup of clam broth into which you have mixed: 2 tbsp. sherry, 2 tbsp. oyster sauce (which you must buy in Chinatown), and 1 tbsp. cornstarch. Stir until the soup thickens.

To make this even more interesting, add 2 tsp. very finely chopped lemon rind and 1 tsp. duck sauce (which you can buy in a Chinese market) or chutney (which you can buy anywhere).

Codfish Soup

This is less spectacular than the two mixed seafood soups, but far simpler and more economical.

Ingredients:

1 lb. fillet of cod
2 tbsp. corn oil margarine
¼ tsp. sweet basil
½ small onion, chopped
2 tsp. Worcestershire sauce
1 C. clam broth
2 C. skimmed milk
salt
pepper

Steam the cod fillet in a wire vegetable steamer for about fifteen minutes, or until you can flake it with a fork.

In a saucepan, melt the margarine; add the basil, the onion, the Worcestershire sauce, and the clam broth. Bring swiftly to a boil, turn the flame to low, and pour in the skimmed milk. Add salt and pepper (preferably white pepper) to taste.

When this begins to simmer add the codfish, which you have separated into individual flakes with a fork.

As soon as it simmers, serve immediately.

This goes well with boiled potatoes and buttered carrots.

Another Soup with Cod

Ingredients:

2 or 3 medium-sized onions, chopped fine
2 tbsp. vegetable oil
1 lb. fillet of cod
2 C. clam broth or water
Tabasco sauce
½ tsp. ground nutmeg
salt

Sauté the onions in the vegetable oil. When they are lightly brown, pour off the fat.

Put the cod fillet into a saucepan and pour in the clam broth or water. Add onions, plus a splash of Tabasco sauce, the nutmeg, and some salt. Boil gently for about fifteen minutes.

Serve in a warm soup tureen.

ESPECIALLY FOR
VEGETARIANS

Mulligatawny Soup

Here's an unusual, easy-to-make soup from India which
vegetarians will like.

Ingredients:

1 C. dried lentils
8 C. water
2 vegetable bouillon cubes
2 tbsp. corn oil margarine
2 cloves garlic, crushed
½ C. onions, finely chopped
1 tsp. salt
Tabasco sauce
3 level tsp. curry powder
lime or lemon juice

Pick over the lentils and throw away the few that
look strange. Rinse the rest and put them in a saucepan
with the water and bouillon cubes. Cover and simmer
for an hour.

About ten minutes before the hour is up, melt the
margarine in a frying pan; add the garlic and onions.
Stir this over a medium flame for five minutes, then add
the salt, Tabasco sauce and curry powder. Stir for a
minute and add to the lentils. Simmer for half an hour.

Puree all this in a blender or force it through a sieve
with a spoon.

The result should be a thin, piquant soup. If it is too
thick, add a little vegetable broth made with another
bouillon cube.

When you serve it, squeeze a little lime or lemon
juice into each serving.

Lentil Casserole

This is a hearty main dish for vegetarians. Leftovers can be served chilled as a side dish.

Ingredients:

1 C. dried lentils
2 C. water
2 vegetable bouillon cubes
3 cloves garlic
½ C. celery, coarsely chopped
2 or 3 green peppers, sliced
4 medium-sized onions, sliced
1½ C. tomato sauce
1 tsp. curry powder
2 tbsp. lemon juice
1 tbsp. soy sauce
Tabasco sauce
1 C. parsley, chopped

Pick over the lentils and throw away the few that look strange.

Soak the lentils in water for an hour. Drain, and simmer them in the water with the bouillon cubes and garlic for about 45 minutes.

In another pan steam the celery, peppers, and onions. Add these to the lentils along with the tomato sauce, curry powder, lemon juice, soy sauce, and 2 or 3 good dashes of Tabasco.

Heat. Just before serving add the parsley.

Beets and Their Tops

Beets have a gentle, inoffensive flavor, though few people (I know of none) develop any strong fondness for them. Borscht, or beet soup, is something else; we'll come to that later.

As I mentioned in an earlier chapter, there is a chemical in beets useful to brain functioning. They are not particularly rich in vitamins, though the greens have lots of vitamin A and calcium. Therefore, let's boil some beets along with their tops. Young beets are best. They are small and firm and their leaves, which wilt quickly, should be fresh.

There is a trick to boiling them. They bleed. When this happens their color and taste escape. Therefore, rinse them in cold water, then cut off the greens 2 inches from the tops of the beets. Be careful not to injure the skins of the beets themselves. Now cut away and discard the lower parts of the stems from the leaves. These are tough.

Ingredients:

1 bunch young, small beets with their leaves
(about 8 beets)
1 C. boiling water with 1 tsp. salt added
2 tbsp. corn oil margarine
1 tbsp. lemon juice
white pepper (optional)

Put the beets in a pot, then add the greens. Pour the boiling water over them and boil, covered, for 15 minutes.

Pour off the water, rinse the beets in cold water until they are cool enough to handle, and skin them.

Melt the margarine, add the beets, greens, and lemon. Reheat, and serve, with a dash of white pepper, if you wish.

This is enough for about 4 servings.

Beet Soup, or Borscht

Ingredients:

1 bunch young, small beets with their tops
(about 8 beets)
3 tbsp. onion, finely chopped
2 tbsp. lemon juice
1 pt. sour cream
chopped parsley

Boil the beets and their tops as in the previous recipe. Set aside the tops and serve them with margarine and lemon as a side dish.

Put the beets through a dicer or blender and add them to the fluid left from boiling them.

Add the onion.

Boil for about a minute, then add the lemon juice.

Pour into 3 soup bowls. On each serving, float 3 tbsp. of sour cream and a pinch of parsley.

This can be served cold if you prefer. Chill the soup in the refrigerator, then add the sour cream and parsley just before serving.

Beets in a Raw Vegetable Salad

Ingredients:

2 small young beets
2 medium-sized carrots
½ Spanish onion
2 celery stalks
6 cherry tomatoes
6 lettuce leaves
black pepper
salad dressing

Grate the beets and carrots. Finely chop the onion and celery. Cut each tomato into quarters. Tear the lettuce leaves into bite-sized pieces. Add a dash of pepper and mix it all up. Serve with whatever salad dressing you choose.

Spinach in Anchovy Sauce

If you have trouble convincing children to eat spinach, this recipe may prove to be the breakthrough:

Ingredients:

1½ lb. spinach
3 tbsp. peanut oil
3 cloves garlic, crushed
1 medium onion, sliced thin
¼ tsp. dried chili peppers
2 anchovy fillets, chopped fine (optional)
1 tbsp. water

Rinse the spinach thoroughly and tear the leaves into bite-sized pieces.

Heat the peanut oil in a frying pan; add the garlic, onion, chili peppers, and anchovies. Pile on the spinach, add the water, and cover. Cook over moderate heat for only five minutes, stirring once.

Eggplant, Chinese Style

Ingredients:

2 lb. eggplant
4 tbsp. peanut oil
3 cloves garlic, crushed
½ C. water
2 tbsp. soy sauce

Wash and peel the eggplant, then cut it into one-inch cubes.

Into a large, very hot frying pan pour the oil and add the garlic. Stir the garlic around for a minute and discard it.

Fry the eggplant for two minutes, then add the water and soy sauce. Cover and simmer for about 15 minutes.

Mushrooms

Mushrooms are too often simply added to something else. There is no need for them to play only a supporting role—they can do quite well in solo parts. Here are three ways:

Mushrooms with Lemon

Ingredients:

1 lb. mushrooms
5 tbsp. corn oil margarine
3 tbsp. lemon juice
¼ tsp. powdered nutmeg
½ tsp. cornstarch (optional)

Rinse the mushrooms, snap off the stems, and cut away the discolored bottoms. If they are large mushrooms, you may want to cut the caps into 2 or 3 pieces.

Use a frying pan or saucepan with a tight cover. Melt the margarine and add all ingredients except the cornstarch. Cover and cook over a moderate flame for about 10 minutes. Thicken the sauce with cornstarch, if you wish, and serve.

Mushrooms Sautéed with Marsala

This is a variation on the above. Eliminate the lemon juice and nutmeg, and instead use ¼ tsp. sweet basil and 2 tbsp. Marsala.

Mushrooms Stuffed with Mushrooms

This is a variation on either of the above two recipes. You'll need large mushrooms for this one.

Finely chop the stems and cook them either with lemon juice or Marsala. Reduce the cooking time to 3 minutes.

Put the cooked mushroom stems into the raw caps, along with about a teaspoon of the sauce, and broil 6 inches from the flame for about 10 minutes.

AFTERWORD
BY PHILIP MIELE

This book stems from a division of labor: Dr. Frank is author of all the ideas in it; I am the writer of all the sentences. I put myself to this task because I believe Dr. Frank is one of the most significant persons on the "medical" scene today. He is searching—successfully, I believe—for very basic, natural ways of curing disease and keeping us healthy. He needed a writer simply because he is too busy with these more important things.

Now I shall intrude on this book for the first time with a few observations of my own.

As we proceeded from one draft to another, and then to another and still another, Dr. Frank's conservatism kept leading to more and more toning down of the descriptions of the results of his work. Words like "spectacular" were reduced to "significant." Phrases like "highly significant" survived only after long discussions. But more important, he has allowed few references to the sacrifices he makes to carry on his research.

This nation rewards its physicians well. They are well housed, they drive expensive cars, and they don't have to skimp on their vacations. Most of them are hardworking and conscientious, but they are damned well off.

Dr. Frank lives in Spartan simplicity. He can afford no vacations; he owns no car. How materially different his life would be if he practiced medicine the way most of our physicians do!

Money is rarely the spur that puts really creative scientists to work. But they do want to live in the society of their professional fellows and be recognized for their accomplishments. This is largely denied to Dr. Frank.

His scientific papers, though submitted, are not published in the medical journals nor presented at medical meetings. There is no conscious conspiracy against him; it is simply the way the system works. Scientists, as anyone interested in the history of science knows, are not hospitable to radical ideas which shake the underpinnings of their life's work.

The word radical, by the way, makes Dr. Frank cringe. He is conservative (from my perspective, almost to the point of eccentricity), and is comfortable with the word only when it is used, as I use it here, in its very strictest sense. The word, like the word radish, comes from a Latin word meaning *root*. A radical idea then is one that deals with the very root of the matter, not its mere appearances.

Dr. Frank's spectacular findings stem from truly radical thought. He is obviously working with something very close to the root cause of health and disease—a way of dealing safely with the renewable energy of the living cells.

There is another sense, however, in which he is profoundly conservative. He is convinced that nature is logical in all ways. No exceptions. There is nothing unusual about this; it is a faith that underlies all scientific enquiry. "I shall never believe that God plays dice with the world," was Albert Einstein's memorable way of saying the same thing.

Beyond this, I discern in Dr. Frank a similarly deep conviction that nature is benign, on our side. Do things nature's way and you have something powerful going for you. Depart from nature, and terrible things must be printed after the word "caution" on medicine bottles.

This kind of conservatism leads, paradoxically, to unorthodox ways of searching out the truth. His basic research starts in his head and remains there throughout much of the process. Experimental work comes much later than in most medical research. For Dr. Frank, the experiment is more a demonstration of what he has already learned through logical thought, and less a way of gathering new information. Of course, he repeats his experiments often enough to average out whatever differences there may be between one laboratory animal and another, and is then content that his findings are either "significant" or not.

Remember, he deals with nutrients and extracts of them that are natural to the body, not with powerful drugs which might show life-ruining side effects in one or two cases out of a thousand. This sharply reduces his need for experiments in giant numbers. The difference between the way he works and the way most medical researchers work has, I believe, something to do with why his findings remain unpublished by established journals.

He is not totally without public recognition, however. He is credited with being the "originator of nucleic-acid therapy" in *Slowing Down the Aging Process* (New York: Pyramid Publications, 1973), a widely read book by Hans J. Kugler, Ph. D. Dr. Kugler is also a medical researcher in the field of aging.

The results of Dr. Frank's work, however, are finding a kind of publication far richer in meaning than printed pages in scientific journals: in the younger-looking faces of his once-elderly patients; in clear, smooth faces once ugly with acne; in the springing steps of patients who only a short time ago were able painfully to plod the length of little more than a city block.

Results of the kind Dr. Frank has achieved with hundreds of patients cannot be ignored forever. Even the most orthodox medical scientist will eventually have to come to terms with a simple, safe therapy which makes so many of the old younger and the sick well. Before that time comes, as Dr. Frank said early in this book, the barricades will be up and the arguments will be fierce. This, he believes, cannot happen too soon.

A few words now about Dr. Frank, the man. He belongs to no associations, has no hobbies, both for the same reason: He has no time.

He is tall, erect, and slim, and has a gentle face that

is strangely ambiguous about his age. It is too mature to be youthful, too smooth and well colored to be old. I asked and learned that he was born May 3, 1923, in Mount Kisco, New York.

His education includes a degree in mathematics from New York University, studies at the University of Fribourg and his medical degree from the University of Geneva, both in Switzerland. He has been in medical practice in New York since 1963, with a brief interruption in the early seventies when he directed a medical research team in Portugal.

I said earlier that I decided to work with Dr. Frank on this book because I believe him to be one of the most significant persons on the medical scene today. That belief was necessary but not enough. I had to know if, in the months ahead, I could work comfortably with him.

One filthy winter day, he and I were struggling against the wind on a Manhattan street. He was dressed in a suit with his jacket open; I was in a heavy coat and muffler. We were chiding each other for our political views, as we still do. I had just said something unacceptably leftish about poverty and he said:

"Whenever I walk these streets, I think about the poor souls behind all those windows who have to go through life locked up in sick bodies. That," he said, paralleling my comment on poverty, "just isn't necessary."

I knew I could work with the man.

Philip Miele

Appendix I

A Molecular Basis of Aging

The process limiting the maximal life span of any species, including man, has not yet been elucidated. This of course appears to have a different basis from that group of processes which cause individual life spans to vary among members of any given species. It is the latter to which we have earlier addressed ourselves in this book. The author would like to propose a theory that may help explain the general nature of aging in man and other species of animals.

It is known that the life spans of animals vary more or less inversely with their characteristic rates of metabolism, and any interspecies theory of aging will have to consider this basic fact. Work has already been done which has shown that immature animals given a diet low in tryptophane have arrested development and slowed aging. They can, however, develop cataracts, as was seen in rodents by Albanese in 1942. Recently, Segal at Berkeley has extended these observations. It has also been observed that these animals age normally when later placed on a diet which also contains normal amounts of tryptophane. Ichihara in Japan observed that quinonimine carboxylic acid, isolated from the urine of patients with senile cataracts, when injected into guinea pigs caused cataracts in a very high percentage of animals. This compound and many others related to it are believed to be derivatives of 5-hydroxykynurenine and 5-hydroxyanthranilic acid, both uncommon tryptophane metabolites found in chicken urine and perhaps in human urine. Price and Brown synthesized a compound, the hydroxylamine derivative of 5-hydroxyanthranilic acid. This compound has not yet been isolated from vertebrate urine or blood. Many other compounds of this type, many of them suggestive of a quinone-related nucleus, actual or potential, undoubtedly exist in vertebrate metabolism, though very small in concentration with respect to the concentration of the usual tryptophane metabolites. They may be synthesized by enzymes structurally related to those in the more usual tryptophane pathways. Such enzymes may become more activated under certain circumstances, as in aging, which in some instances also leads to cataract formation. Degenerative changes resulting from oxidative and other noxious, fortuitous processes may initially trigger these activations of originally quiescent enzymes. Such initiation of enzyme activation may involve DNA alterations at some point.

It is also known that homogentisic acid can make an oxidation-reduction (redox) system with benzoquinone acetic acid. These are both related derivatives of tyrosine metabolism. The latter compound has been found in the urine of vitamin-deficient guinea pigs (Fishberg, Ichihara). Homogentisic acid prolongs the survival of animals with scurvy, and probably this is related to the particular dihydroxyl nature of both compounds. The related compound benzoquinone acetic acid caused cataracts in animals previously on a low-ascorbic-acid diet for one week; this was prevented by the administration of ascorbic acid. These compounds of course can form redox systems when paired. Of interest here also is the similarity of these compounds structurally to quinones, particularly the tyrosine derivatives. The frequency of cataracts in older animals and man particularly should also be considered here. It should also be noted that tyrosine is a precursor of the quinone ring of ubiquinone (coenzyme Q) by way of, successively, parahydroxyphenyllactic acid, parahydroxybenzoic acid, 5-dimethoxyubiquinone-9 and finally ubiquinone-9. The long side chain of coenzyme Q is derived from multiples of isoprene groups, which are early metabolites on the main pathway in the chain of compounds involved in cholesterol synthesis. Also to be considered are the often-raised cholesterol levels of older people.

It is the author's contention that all these seemingly diverse reactions are importantly and metabolically related.

Coenzyme Q is an extremely important link between the energy-giving metabolism in the Krebs cycle, or other energy-giving catabolic pathways which involve energy transfers to NAD (nicotinamide adenine dinucleotide) and FAD (flavin adenine dinucleotide), and the energy- or electron-carrying enzymes of the electron transfer chain. These latter units of course transfer their energy to the final energy-carrying compound, adenosine triphosphate (ATP). Clearly, any influence which diminishes the synthesis or function of coenzyme Q will diminish the energy level of the involved cells in the body. It is the author's contention that quinonimine carboxylate or other compounds derived from 5-hydroxykynurenine or 5-hydroxyanthranilic acid, or related compounds of tryptophane metabolism, because of their quinonelike nature or potential, interfere with the action of the quinone, coenzyme Q, or its synthesis. These compounds have a similarity to the reduced form of coenzyme Q, except that a carboxyl group replaces the methyl group of coenzyme Q and one hydroxyl group of coenzyme Q is replaced by nitrogen-containing groups which may be converted to carbonyl or hydroxyl groups. The imine groups can of course be converted to carbonyl groups. One or more of these compounds may metabolically partially replace coenzyme Q, so that the latter's activity is much reduced. The enzyme specificities of those enzymes involved with coenzyme Q are not known too well. The tyrosine metabolite, homogentisic acid, does structurally resemble reduced coenzyme Q, but in this instance the methyl group of coenzyme Q is replaced by an acetyl group ortho to a hydroxyl group. Coenzyme Q also has two methoxy groups on the quinone ring, but it is possible that these are also formed on hydroxylated derivatives of 5-hydroxyanthranilic acid or its related metabolites, though such a correspondence may not be critical. Certainly, the pathways of tryptophane metabolism or the enzyme specificities involved in this area have not been explored sufficiently. The example given of the partial substitution of homogentisic acid-benzoquinone acetic acid for vitamin C show functionally how such compounds may operate.

Though cataracts appear in animals on a low tryptophane diet and also in those given quinonimine carboxylic acid, it would seem that such trypotophane metabolites occur as a result of the activation of normally somewhat unusual or aberrant metabolic pathways. Such activated pathways would occur in the lens with low or very low tryptophane intake. These unusual or relatively inactive metabolic pathways can become more activated in aging as well, as was earlier mentioned. Many of the changes in cataracts are suggestive of changes in aging in related tissues. The lens has a low rate of energy metabolism, and coenzyme Q is present in relatively small amounts. If inactivated functionally, it would transfer even less energy for the continuation of the function of lens tissue. Very possibly, by the mechanism suggested, coenzyme Q is critically inactivated preliminary to senile cataract formation, and the lens tissue is then gradually and pathologically altered. It is significant that uncoupling agents, which interfere with energy transfer to ATP, also have caused cataracts.

One important mechanism of cataract formation stresses the importance of polyols (dulcitol, sorbitol) in their formation. These compounds would increase osmotic pressure and subsequent precipitation of celular proteins, etc. The decrease in activity of coenzyme Q here described, even though the lens has a low Krebs-cycle metabolism, would gradually lead to increased levels of NADH (reduced NAD). Also involved in the oxidation of NADH is glycerophosphate dehydrogenase, which converts dihydroxyacetone phosphate to glycerol 3-phosphate. This latter compound carries the NADH into mitochondria where it would be oxidized by coenzyme Q. The raised NADH levels would have this origin. These would lead to increased levels of NADPH (reduced NAD phosphate) by one of the transhydrogenase mechanisms, and the increased NADPH would activate polyol dehydrogenase, bringing about the synthesis of polyols. Though decreased activity of pentose-shunt metabolism has been described in cataractous lenses, this may be brought about by inhibition of 6-phosphogluconate dehydrogenase by the increased NADPH. The net balance probably favors an increased level of NADPH. The lens does have a relatively significant requirement for ATP synthesis, because it is needed for glutathione synthesis as well as for other synthesis. A purely anaerobic metabolism would probably not provide enough of ATP, especially if glycolysis were inhibited, as it is by galactose-1 phosphate. The enzymes of the citric-acid cycle are present, but low in activity. Similar processes would explain the various corneal dysplasias found in older people. The retina, which has the highest oxygen consumption of any body tissue, would clearly be affected by the reduced coenzyme Q activity. This would explain the incidence of senile macular degeneration in older people. Glutathione (reduced) is of course important for reducing peroxides, and so on, and NADPH serves to reduce glutathione. These peroxides, and so on, may be crucial in protein changes and cataract formation.

In aging per se, there may be a gradual buildup of one or more of these quinonelike compounds of tryptophane, and perhaps of tyrosine metabolism as well. The(se) compound(s) would more and more antimetabolically deactivate coenzyme Q, or interfere with its synthesis by metabolically "replacing" its near precursor(s). One illustration of a possible mechanism for interference with the synthesis of coenzyme Q would involve the coenzyme Q precursor, parahydroxybenzoic acid or a more proximate compound, in a "pseudosubstrate" reaction similar to that shown in the interference with the hydroxylation of salicylic acid by salicylate hydroxylase, which is produced by benzoic acid, the pseudosubstrate. In this latter case, hydrogen peroxide is produced instead of a hydroxylated salicylic acid. Though this particular mechanism may not occur with coenzyme Q synthesis, it illustrates in a general fashion how one compound may interfere with another in this synthetic process. In young animals or man, there would be a very low level of these "abnormal" metabolites, which would build up in time; and this buildup and its triggering would be caused by degenerative processes occurring with time in all living things because of oxidative reactions and other types of degradative processes as described earlier. The buildup of these continually occurring degradative processes would of course be enhanced by the simultaneous increase of the coenzyme-Q-interfering metabolites referred to. The two sets of processes would be mutually reinforcing. Also, the removal of these noxious tryptophane (or tyrosine) metabolite(s) would be increasingly interfered with for perhaps similar reasons, so that more and more, these two sets of processes would reinforce each other. Here, the dominant process would probably become that related to coenzyme Q. Indeed, as the animal aged more and more, the energy-depleting dysfunction or nonfunction of coenzyme Q would become so dominant that the animal body would ultimately cease functioning. The many other metabolic malfunctions brought about variously by other sources of degeneration, dietary and otherwise, would also be critical and massive. It would appear reasonable to assume that animals with a faster rate of metabolism and hence a shorter life span would be those having a potentially greater rate of production of these coenzyme-Q-interfering metabolites. They would also have a far greater need for oxygen and coenzyme Q, and for this reason they would have shorter life spans.

That the removal rates generally of these noxious metabolites may tend to be slower, in relative terms, than their buildup could be because of intrinsically present enzymic processes. These would be aided by degradative processes from oxidative and other degenerative events. Kidney and eliminative function would also be increasingly impaired for these reasons. But even here, an increased rate of synthesis of the energy-depleting tryptophane metabolite(s), and a constant eliminative rate, would be all that would be needed for an increasing negative effect on coenzyme Q.

Mention was made before of raised cholesterol levels in those who are older. It was also mentioned that the side chain of coenzyme Q is provided by isoprene groups on the pathway to cholesterol synthesis. Cholesterol synthesis involves the following compounds in sequence, briefly: acetyl coenzyme A (Co A), acetoacetyl Co A, beta hydroxy beta methylglutaryl Co A, mevalonic acid, delta 3 isopentenyl pyrophosphate (the isoprene group), squalene, lanosterol, cholesterol. The isoprene group can also become the side chain of coenzyme Q and the cytochrome oxidase porphyrin and other compounds. The control mechanism determining which way it goes is not known. Reference was made to diminished function or synthesis of coenzyme Q resulting from the quinone-related metabolites of tryptophane or tyrosine. Thus, the lower level or turnover rate of coenzyme Q would result in less demand for isoprene groups to form its side chain and would, further, lead to a greater activity of the cholesterol pathway from the delta 3 isopentenyl pyrophosphate compound. An important influence on cholesterol synthesis in older people would relate to decreased oxidation of acetyl Co A because of the compromised Co Q blockage of the Krebs cycle and oxidative metabolism. What ATP is available from the anaerobic glycolysis preceding acetyl Co A formation, and such that is available from the reduced aerobic metabolism, would more readily be used in the buildup of cholesterol in the sequence before described, beginning with acetyl Co A. NADPH levels, important in cholesterol and fat synthesis, are also raised. In particular, the fats which would be oxidized to acetyl Co A, as well as the acetyl Co A formed from the amino acids, would not be as readily further oxidizable by way of the Krebs cycle and the electron transport chain. In such a situation, triglycerides could form, but cholesterol synthesis would be more readily produced as well. Those fats in a more reduced form would be less completely oxidized than those fats which are less reduced because the Co Q blockage point would be more inhibiting in the case of the former compound's larger number of necessary oxidative steps. Such considerations would not only help explain the differences found between the effects of saturated and unsaturated fats on cholesterol levels, but would also help explain why cholesterol levels are higher in older people. Nucleic-acid-rich diets lower cholesterol because they increase ATP formation, enhance electron transport chain activity and Co Q and cytochrome oxidase synthesis, and also increase NADH (NADPH) oxidation (see below).

It is known that there is an increased incidence of cancer in older people. Cancer cells are also known to have a generally lower level of energy than normal cells, and to have predominantly an anaerobic metabolism. One of the important reasons for this type of metabolism could well relate to the herein described deficiencies in Co Q level or function. It is entirely possible that such an anaerobic metabolism would favor cancer formation. It would definitely favor tumor growth.

It has been theorized that the basis of the biological clock is related to a segment of DNA programmed hereditarily for death. The manner of this programming is not defined. The author's hypothesis would relate the decay of DNA seen in aging to a fundamental decrease in the energy (ATP) needed for DNA repair. This would be aided by simultaneous degeneration based on oxidative and other nonprogrammed processes. The union of both sets of processes would result in increasing and generalized metabolic dysfunction. Important, however, in the author's hypothesis, is the triggering and continuation of those particular enzymic actions leading to the Co-Q-limiting compound(s) described. Whether the basis of this directly or resultantly lies in the DNA, and whether such is exquisitely or singularly programmed, cannot be stated yet. Such an assumption, though, is unnecessary.

Reference was made in earlier publications* by the author to the antianoxia and also to the antiaging effects of exogenous nucleic acids. A part of the antianoxia effect gotten with nucleic acids would result from an enhanced Co Q synthesis, which would involve increases in the synthesis of the enzymes concerned in this process, and also increased levels and turnover rates of ATP; this would also favorably influence Co Q synthesis. Co Q would tend to help maximize the processes involved in the subsequent steps of the electron transport chain, resulting in more efficient oxygen utilization and greater energy formation, in the nature of more efficient ATP synthesis. Of course, as described earlier, the function of nucleic acids in connection with oxygen utilization efficiency may similarly involve a more efficient basis for the synthesis of the other units in the electron transport chain as well, and also as described, bring about an increased number of more properly formed mitochondria. These would also carry more Co Q, as well as more of the other normally formed units in the electron transport chain. Cytochrome oxidase would thus also be increased. Since it has a Vmax with a low partial pressure of oxygen at 4 to 5 mmHg, more of the available oxygen would be used to capture elec-

* (1) Frank, B., *A New Approach to Degenerative Disease and Aging*. N.Y.: Patria Press, 1964. (2) Frank, B., *Nucleic Acid Therapy of Aging and Degenerative Disease*. 3rd ed. Lisbon: Fiquima, 1975. (3) Unpublished papers and correspondence, 1961–64.

trons. This oxygen would be readily replenished each time the blood passes through the lungs, but with each cycle a greater proportion of oxygen would be used than would be usual. Such an increased usage of oxygen would be most salutary in aging. It is these considerations which show the relation of increased nucleic-acid intake to the process here described involving Co Q and other electron-transport chain units in aging. The converse situation, with decreased nucleic-acid intake, can also be explained by a related reasoning.

The author believes that the processes here described, relating tryptophane and tyrosine metabolism to Co Q, as well as that described relating to cytochrome oxidase, form the molecular basis for the aging of species. It is also obvious that the variations between different animal species in their life spans could well result from differences in the nature of the enzymes involved in the formation, fate, and function of tryptophane and tyrosine metabolites which relate to the quinones and Co Q, and possibly to other processes relating to cytochrome oxidase. The hypothesis would appear to have both plausibility and relative simplicity. It should not be difficult to test out this hypothesis and to devise appropriate dietary and metabolic corrections for the aberrant compound or compounds involved. Administration of Co Q or its precursors is one apparent possibility. Other, better possibilities would involve selective diversion of the metabolic pathways involved in the synthesis of deleterious trytophane or tyrosine derivatives. Other amino acids (aromatic or otherwise) must also be considered, as well as other metabolites which could form such Co-Q-inhibiting compounds. Those involved with tryptophane or tyrosine metabolism appear the most promising to the author. There are some who believe that menaquinone is involved in the electron transport chain. If it is, a somewhat similar reasoning as that for Co Q might have relevance here. In the aging-retarding sense as well, quinone-related compounds which can function as reversible antioxidants may also play a role. Nicotinamide, because of the inhibition of tryptophane dioxygenase by pyridine nucleotides, offers one initial therapeutic possibility. Supplementation with cytochrome oxidase porphyrin or precursors might also be useful.

Of interest also, in the potential relation of quinones to aging, is the lessened skin aging in those having greatly pigmented skin, i.e. more melanin granules in the basal layer of the epidermis. The melanin procursor is indole 5, 6-quinone, which is derived from tyrosine. Of course, the decreased skin-aging rate of these people is often attributed solely to the screening out of ultraviolet rays from the sun, and this has already been alluded to in this book. However, the author is curious about the possible relation of indole 5, 6-quinone and ubiquinone, another tyrosine derivative. Though the structures of both compounds differ, and though the active carbonyl groups are ortho and para respectively, there is the possibility that indole 5, 6-quinone may be metabolized further, by a yet unknown pathway. The resulting compound might stimulate the synthesis of ubiquinone or diminish the activity of Co-Q-interfering metabolites of tryptophane. In older Caucasian skin, pigmented areas are often seen in aging. Within this framework, such deposition of melanin would presume that the postulated pathway from indole 5, 6-quinone is much less active. Whether these suggested antiaging possibilities involving indole 5, 6-quinone are correct, only further research will determine. There would of course also be the possibility that indole 5, 6-quinone or derivatives could function positively in the place of or in addition to Co Q.

Since the diet of all or nearly all living things involves the taking in of the amino acids tryptophane ad tyrosine nutritionally, or the synthesis of these from other nutrients, it would appear that the mechanism here posited for the control of the various species' life spans offers a common pathway. This hypothesis can rationally explain the various secondary changes known as aging.

Also to be considered are interferences with synthesis or activity of other cytochromes and electron-chain components, as potential incremental factors in energy depletion and aging. The causation of such interferences cannot yet be clarified, and whether energy losses from Co-Q interferences initiate or contribute to these cannot yet be ascertained.

The primal energy-depleting processes described do not enable sufficient repair of the concomitant free radical and oxidatively induced degenerations in DNA and elsewhere in the cell, and thus can be considered the fundamental cause of cellular and corporeal aging. In youth, there is sufficient energy for repair processes.

SUMMARY

It would be useful to summarize this concept of the biological clock in simple terms. It is proposed that fundamentally, the basic process involved in the limitation of the animal life span relates to decreasing energy levels available for metabolic processes in the organism. The origin of this decreasing availability of energy stems from the availability of a key metabolite in the main group of reactions concerned with the absorption and concentration of the energy derived from foodstuffs. This energy is then transmitted in the normal cell to the final energy-carrying molecule, namely adenosine triphosphate (ATP), which fuels virtually all the metabolic reactions in the body. The key compound alluded to here, and critically involved in the energy transfer from food metabolism to ATP, is a quinone compound known as coenzyme Q. This compound is diminished or functionally inhibited in its action during the basic process resulting in aging. This decreased functional level of coenzyme Q is brought about by an interference mediated by the action of one or more coenzyme-Q-like metabolites of the amino acid tryptophane, tyrosine, or other amino acids. Most probably this involves tryptophane.

The trigger mechanism initiating the creation of this coenzyme-Q-interfering metabolite is occasioned by the influence of a compound resulting from the ever-present oxidative or degradative reactions, which result from continually impinging and fortuitous events. Such fortuitous events may relate to cosmic rays, dietary anomalies, or various other environmental toxins. Once the synthesis of coenzyme-Q-interfering metabolite(s) is begun, there is a vicious cycle established between these two sets of processes, and an increasing buildup of the coenzyme-Q-interfering metabolites. The inactivation of coenzyme Q also feeds on itself, so to speak, so that coenzyme Q becomes increasingly inactivated. When advanced aging is reached, the functional capacity of coenzyme Q activity is diminished critically, together with many other metabolic activities including that of the nucleic acids, so that life expires.

Processes involving cytochrome oxidase and other ETC components may play a role as well.

Those species having higher rates of metabolism would produce more of the coenzyme-Q-interfering metabolites of tryptophane, etc., and because they more critically need coenzyme Q would die sooner. Indeed, life spans of animals with higher rates of metabolism are shorter.

Considerations based on the coenzyme-Q-related processes referred to here also explain the basic orgin of much, if not all, of the degeneration seen in aging. Clearly, sufficient energy is needed to carry out normal body functions. Cataracts, higher blood levels of cholesterol, atherosclerosis, atherosclerotic heart disease, cancer, and apparently many other pathological processes of aging can be explained by this theory.

With loss of primal energy in the cell, repair of other

concomitant damage (from free radicals, etc.) cannot occur, as it does in youth.

Because the processes involved are metabolic and related to metabolites of tryptophane, etc., it is anticipated that these will be readily correctable by metabolic means.

Appendix
II

On
Brain Energetics
and Its
Implications

It is well established that the neurons in the brain have a very high rate of oxidative metabolism. The brain receives, at rest, about 20 percent of the oxygen intake of the body and comprises nearly 2 percent of the body weight. This is a result of the brain's, and more particularly the brain neuron's, need for energy in the form of adenosine-5'-triphosphate (ATP). This energy is used in nerve function involving rapid ion fluxes and ATPases. The basic mechanism which insures this high rate of energy and ATP turnover has never been satisfactorily clarified. For this to occur, glucose metabolism through the anaerobic pathway, and the subsequent oxidative phase of metabolism with the Krebs cycle and the electron transport chain, must be relatively unimpeded much of time. It is here proposed that the critical compounds involved in keeping the processes of brain neuronal oxidative metabolism active for this necessary ATP and energy formation are within the family of so-called neuroinhibitors. These include glycine, betaalanine and gamma aminobutyric acid (GABA), N-acetyl aspartic acid, and dopamine. This concept was derived from observations on the effects of these compounds in inhibiting the growth of tumors in mice. This work has been reported elsewhere.[1,2]

Fundamentally the large majority, perhaps all, tumors have a predominant anaerobic metabolism, an observation originally made by Warburg.[4] It has been observed in various experiments on mouse tumors (SA

180, Ehrlich Ca, C3H mammary Ca) that formulations which promote significant Krebs-cycle metabolism in tumors (and host) cause tumor regression. It is the author's view that a fundamental block in achieving aerobic metabolism in tumors lies in the pyruvate dehydrogenase enzyme complex. Associated with this, there is also an overactivity of the enzyme phosphoenolpyruvate carboxykinase, which governs an important control point in gluconeogenesis and subsequent glycolysis. There may also be defects in the electron transport chain and in NADH shuttle mechanisms.

The pyruvate dehydrogenase enzyme complex contains three enzymes: pyruvate decarboxylase, transacetylase, and dihydrolipoyl dehydrogenase, which successively are accompanied by cocarboxylase, lipoic acid, and flavin adenine dinucleotide, as coenzymes. The pyruvate dehydrogenase (pyruvate decarboxylase) is deactivated by a phosphate group transfer from MgATP, by means of a protein kinase attached to the transacetylase component of the enzyme complex. This phosphorylation of the enzyme in turn decreases the activity of pyruvate dehydrogenase, causing an increase in anaerobic metabolism.

It is also known that cyclic AMP increases the activity of phosphoenolpyruvate (PEP) carboxykinase. Reduction of cyclic AMP decreases this activity. Decreased activity of pyruvate dehydrogenase and increased activity of PEP carboxykinase favor tumor growth and decreased oxidative metabolism.

The basic antitumor system was composed of a fuel, glucose or pyruvic acid, the coenzymes of the pyruvate dehydrogenase complex, cocarboxylase, lipoic acid, coenzyme A, flavin adenine dinucleotide (FAD), and nocotinamide adenine dinucleotide (NAD). AMP, ADP and a small amount of ATP, important enzyme modulators favoring Krebs-cycle activity, were also included. With this was included alpha ketoglutaric acid and malic acid, Krebs-cycle metabolites. To this were added varying compounds to increase oxidative metabolism. These included the neuroinhibitors mentioned. This latter group is thought by the author to act by increasing pyruvate dehydrogenase activity.

These formulations were given daily by subcutaneous injection. When this formulation was given without the neuroninhibitors the tumors grew rapidly. Also very active in increasing the growth of these tumors were the components cocarboxylase and lipoic acid, particularly at higher levels; they may thus be involved in inactivating this enzyme at higher levels. Cyclic AMP also caused rapidly increased tumor growth. Cyclic GMP caused inhibition. Octopamine and histamine, which are in the neuroexciter family, when given with the basic formulation caused rapid growth of tumors. These are thought to increase cyclic AMP. When the neuroinhibitors were added varyingly, singly and together, there was tumor inhibition or rapid regression. Pyruvate dehydrogenase activation and possibly alpha ketoglutarate dehydrogenase activation (this enzyme is similar to pyruvate dehydrogenase in its composition) were hypothecated to be critically involved in this tumor regression. PEP carboxykinase inactivation was concluded to be involved in the same dynamic sense.

The author hypothesizes from this and related observations that tumor-growth inhibition involves the rapid and critical decrease of non-mitochondrial-reduced pyridines, which are needed for the various synthetic processes of tumor growth. The apparently increased aerobic metabolism brought about by the neuroinhibitors, which in turn results in increased oxidation of and decreased concentration of reduced pyridines, relates to increased pyruvate dehydrogenase activity. Cytoplasmic NADH formations, in the author's view, is the limiting compound in cell growth.[1,8]

The mature neurons in the brain no longer undergo cell division and are not known to undergo malignant transformation.

For cell division to occur, a relatively large amount of nonmitochondrial* NADH and NADPH are needed for the synthetic processes involved, such as reducing the nucleotides for DNA synthesis, and for the synthesis of lipids and other compounds. (ATP is needed as well for many of these processes, as in the buildup of proteins and purines.) Anaerobic metabolism is more important for dividing cells, where large amounts of reduced pyridines are needed for growth. In brain neurons and mature striated muscle, where relatively large amounts of ATP are needed, the reduced pyridines are largely oxidized to form ATP. The oxidation of NADH is carried out by the electron transport chain, where oxidative metabolism proper occurs. The mitochondrial Krebs cycle is really the forerunner of oxidative metabolism proper, and large amounts of NADH are made here. Lesser but important amounts of reduced pyridines are made in the anaerobic pathway before the pyruvate stage. The dehydrogenase enzymes referred to, as well as PEP carboxykinase, occur at very important control points in the formation of reduced and oxidized pyridines. NAD, also a precursor of NADP, is the pyridine form usually in highest concentration. NADPH, the reduced pyridine used in many syntheses, may be made by transhydrogenation from NADH and also by the phosphogluconate oxidative pathway, which is anaerobic. This latter NADPH-producing pathway begins with the oxidation of glucose-6-phosphate, and occurs before the pyruvate and pyruvate dehydrogenase stage. Inactivation of the latter enzyme would also favor this NADPH-producing pathway, present in neurons and neuroglias.

It is, to repeat, the author's hypothesis that the primary determinant of the occurrence or absence of cell division is critically related to the ratio of reduced to

---

* Brain neurons can also carry on glycolysis in mitochondria, and produce the otherwise nonmitochondrial NADH in mitochondria as well.

oxidized nonmitochondrial* pyridines.[1,3] NADH and NADPH provide the limiting energy for growth processes. Growth-controlling hormones would act ultimately by controlling the levels of the cytoplasmic reduced pyridines. Oxygen-using metabolism, so prominent in the brain and muscle, provides not only ATP but the pyridines are largely oxidized to achieve this. These oxidized pyridines are associated with the arrest of growth.

N-acetyl aspartic acid, seemingly constituted by end-to-end placement of glycine and beta alanine as a double-edged key, is an important neuroinhibitor in the brain. There is a very large concentration in adult cortex, some 5 or more micromoles per gram, and much less in fetal cortex and brain and neuroglias, which are dividing cells. It is enzymatically hydrolyzed to acetate and aspartate in the brain, and is said to function as a donor of acetyl groups for lipid synthesis and as a source of aspartate, a neuroexciter.[5] Probably, however, its primary role is in increasing ATP formation and in limiting nerve-cell division. Aspartate and lipids are represented in converse processes, illustrating nature's parsimony. Dopamine and the other neuroinhibitors would function similarly in limiting nerve cell division and in increasing brain neuron energy production.

Striated muscle, with its high rate of oxidative metabolism, only rarely develops tumors (rhabdomyosarcoma). Beta alanine, a neuroinhibitor, occurs importantly in muscle either alone or in combination with histidine, as carnosine and anserine. Growth-inhibiting processes similar to those in nerves are probably involved in striated muscle, and both brain neurons and striated muscle employ at least partially similar compounds to keep pyruvate and perhaps alpha ketoglutarate dehydrogenase active for an enhanced oxidative metabolism. Both muscle strength and some muscle pathology may relate to this, as in muscular dystrophy.

* See footnote, page 145.

It would be useful to determine beta alanine, carnosine, and anserine levels in this disease, as well as in the muscles of people having varying degrees of strength and endurance.

It appears feasible that cell division of brain and muscle could be stimulated with sufficient increase in the level of reduced pyridines. With appropriate techniques, it may also be possible to achieve control over the degree, rate, and locus of such cell division. In senility, as in cerebrovascular accidents, this would be particularly useful to achieve better brain function, were circulatory problems also ameliorated. The control of senility, however, as a basic aging process would perhaps necessarily and concomitantly also involve some control over the cause of aging.[1,2] Of interest here is the recent report by Davison et al[6] that the activities of L-dopa decarboxylase and glutamic acid decarboxylase, important for the formation of dopamine and GABA, were decreased some 70 to 90 percent in brains with senile dementia. Since these latter compounds appear so important for brain energy, the biochemical lesion in senile brains may partially involve a critical loss of energy from a defect in the accumulation of these compounds, which appear important in the formation of ATP. Of course, such a defect would ultimately lead to loss of brain neurons. Parkinson's disease, with a loss of neurons of the nigro-striatal pathway, may for similar energetic reasons be related to decreased dopamine.

Another area of fundamental importance concerns animal and human intelligence. Various theories have been proposed relating this to the number and complexity of neuronal interconnections in the brain. There does appear to be some relation in brains representing the extremes of intelligence, but in cases of seemingly normal brains, such differences in structure have not been clearly delineated. Energetic differences in brains are probably also an important determinant of intellectual differences. Underlying these may be the activities of various neuroinhibitors, and perhaps other compounds increasing oxidative metabolism. Neuroexcitors would appear to function primarily in the syntheses promoting neuronal interconnection complexity. The neuroglias, being dividing cells, may also be significant providers of reduced pyridines (or their surrogates or carriers) and other compounds needed for syntheses. From this, it is apparent that morphologic changes underlying intelligence may be primarily related to the less oxidative metabolism of neuroglias, and in the same sense to some neuroexcitors, including glutamic and aspartic acids. Such metabolic processes are more prominent in the growing fetal brain. In the adult brain, with a given and relatively stable structure, intelligence may be more critically related to the oxidative neuronal metabolism promoted by the neuroinhibitors.

Pyruvate dehydrogenase activity is most critical for oxidative metabolism. The neuroinhibitors may have an important action in the promotion of the activity of this enzyme.

The fundamental actions of neuroinhibitors in the brain are probably related to increasing brain oxidative metabolism, thereby limiting brain neuronal cell division on the one hand and increasing neuronal activity and intelligence on the other.

BIBLIOGRAPHY

1. Frank B., *Nucleic Acid Therapy of Aging and Degenerative Disease*, 3rd ed. Lisbon: Fiquima, 1975.
2. Frank, B., *A New Approach to Degenerative Disease and Aging*. New York: Patria Press, 1964.
3. Personal communications, 1973, 1974.
4. Warburg, O., "The Causes of Cancer," *Colloq. Ges. Physiol. Chem.*, 1966 (17), pp. 1–16.
5. Reichelt and Kvamme, "Acetylated and Peptide

Bound Glutamate and Aspartate in Brain," *Journal of Neurochemistry,* 1967, pp. 14, 987.

6. Davison, A. N., et al., "Brain Decarboxylase Activities as Indices of Pathological Change in Senile Dementia," *Lancet,* 1974, p. 1247.

Appendix
III

On
Biologic
Degeneration

From the many observations and ideas described, the author hypothesizes that most degenerative disease is critically related to the balance between oxidative and nonoxidative metabolism. Degenerative pathology is fundamentally caused by an enduring abnormal increase or predominance in critical tissues of anaerobic over aerobic metabolism. Such an increase is brought about by continuing changing in the enzyme functions needed for proper oxidative metabolism. This situation reduces ATP energy and increases cytoplasmic-reduced pyridines, and results in diminished cell function and repair, as well as in an abnormal growth of critical tissues or in the synthesis of abnormal compounds and structures. This latter constitutes the basic pathology of degenerative disease.

The growth of cancer has already been related to a decrease in pyruvate dehydrogenase activity, with possibly associated blockages in the electron transport chain and the malate aspartate and other shuttle mechanisms, as well as an overactivity of PEP carboxykinase because of increased cyclic AMP. This results in an increase of glycolysis and reduced pyridines and growth, as well as of lactic acid, which serves as a reservoir for reduced pyridines. Normal growth was also described as being critically dependent on the level of cytoplasmic-reduced pyridines.

In diabetes millitus, inhibition of pyruvate dehydrogenase and other alpha keto decarboxylase enzymes, because of defects in the formation of thiamine pyrophosphate, and perhaps of coenzyme A and other coenzymes of the B complex, is most critical. The higher glucose levels, with the resulting increase in levels of reduced pyridines, occasion the synthesis of the thickened and abnormal arteriolar basement membrane layer, which is the pathological hallmark of this disease. Nucleic acid intake, which increases the rate of ATP formation, is a most essential component of therapy. Because of the interference in the Krebs-Szent-Györgyi cycle gateway and in normal ATP production, the alpha glycerophosphate shuttle may be overactive as an energy source. This in turn decreases the synthesis of certain lipids, particularly phospholipids, and brings about the nerve defects of diabetic neuropathy, as well as other cellular abnormalities. This conclusion prompted the author to administer five or more grams daily of magnesium glycerophosphate (choline and inositol, alone, were of little use in such severe cases [4]) with good improvement. The magnesium glycerophosphate was associated with B complex, choline, inositol, and other factors already mentioned as useful in this condition, but which were no longer very effective.*

---

* The primary role of glycerophosphate relates here to cell membrane and membranelle formation, i.e., phospholipid synthesis. More recent work by the author has shown that magnesium glycerophosphate intake produced good improvement in chronic hepatitis, presbyopia and other degenerative conditions involving cell membrane pathology, including an increase in dermal smoothness.

Cell membrane pathology, in the author's view, arises mainly from the decrease in oxidative metabolism in cells undergoing degeneration. This is brought about by the increased oxidation of glycerophosphate, as was described in the case of diabetic neuropathy, because it provides an alternative pathway, from anaerobic metabolism, for the production of ATP. In diabetic neuropathy the block in aerobic metabolism is brought about by an abnormal metabolism of thiamine and perhaps other B vitamins, whereas the block in other conditions and aging involves other processes, such as those involving the electron transport chain and other points. This may in some instances include the B vitamins as well.

The relation of hypercholesteremia and atherosclerosis to defects in oxidative metabolism and electron transport chain activity, as well as the related defects in aging, were already explained. The relation of nucleic-acid-rich diets to the lowering of cholesterol because of increased ATP turnover, enhanced electron transport chain activity with greater coenzyme Q and cytochrome oxidase synthesis (which shifts isoprene metabolism from cholesterol formation), and also the associated increased NADH (NADPH) oxidation, was mentioned as important in the therapy of atherosclerosis, as well as in its prevention. Increased dolichol phosphate synthesis with diets richer in nucleic acids would play a similar role, as dolichols are isoprenoid compounds.

One interesting problem in the pathology of carcinoid syndrome will serve as a typical example of the utility of this approach to degenerative disease. This is the problem of origin of the mucopolysaccharide accretion on, and narrowing of, the right atrioventricular heart valve. The liver metastases of serotonin-producing cells bring about a large secretion of serotonin, a neuroexcitor, mostly concentrated in the venous blood pouring on this valve. Most, if not all, neuroexcitors inhibit oxidative metabolism, increase gluconeogenesis, and reduced pyridines and synthetic processes. The converse occurs with the neuroinhibitors. It may thus be readily understood how mucopolysaccharides accumulate on the right heart valve.

Many other phenomena lend themselves to this ap-

Because of the increased destruction, via oxidation, of that fraction of glycerophosphate normally used for phospholipid synthesis, there is a lessened synthesis of phospholipids. The apparently increased need of dietary essential fatty acids (cis-cis linoleic and arachidonic acids, for example) in certain degenerative conditions and diabetes may also relate to this because of the increased availability of these fatty acids, needed for phospholipid synthesis, would help utilize that glycerophosphate available. The same would apply to other constituents of phospholipids.

proach, and will be described in a forthcoming book. The giant size of dinosaurs, and later mammals of the tertiary period of the earth, when the oxygen levels of the atmosphere were much lower, is not a mere coincidence, nor was the very small size of the earliest mammals of the Mesozoic era, when oxygen levels were too low for significant growth of these early warm-blooded creatures. The author believes that slow evolutionary adaptation with a more dominant anaerobic, growth-producing metabolism was of critical influence in the former.

The larger size of younger people in the modern Western world has an abstractedly similar causation, but the operative mechanisms are very different. Here the lower oxidative metabolism is brought about by oxidative metabolism enzyme poisons, in the nature of pollutants, toxins, drugs, and various chemicals used in food growth and preparation, with an associated increase in intake of carbohydrates and a decrease in dietary nucleic acids. The decreasing levels of atmospheric oxygen resulting from forest destruction and sea pollution will play an increasing potentiating role. This pattern is also the basis for most modern degenerative disease in the Western world.

The gigantism observed in species prior to their disappearance can probably be explained by a related reasoning.

In sum, evolution of the human species in the optimal sense is likely no longer progressing, but on the contrary is very probably regressing. Fortunately, this dark tide can be reversed.

Index

Fats, 8, 9, 87; foods high in saturated, 79; unsaturated, 73, 79

Fatty acids, 8

Fertilizer, chemical vs. organic, 43

Fish, 41-42, 44, 61, 73; amino acids in, 96, 129; canned vs. fresh, 105; Chinese cooking of, 130-132; 136; selecting fresh, 129; size of, and pollutants, 101; vegetarians and, 96-97

Fish recipes, 130-137; cassoulet with salmon, 132-133; codfish soup, 136-137; mixed seafood soup, Chinese style, 136; mixed seafood soup, Mediterranean style, 135; salmon chowder, 133-135; steamed, in black bean sauce, 130-132

Frank, Dr. Benjamin, 7, 8, 10, 145-148

Free radicals and oxidative processes: as cause of aging and degenerative disease, 109

Fructose, 8

Fruits, 96; juices, 42, 92, 97

Galactose, 8

Gangrene, 85

Gelatin, unflavored, 86

Glaucoma, 116

Glucose, 8, 87

Glycerol, 8, 87; phosphate, 111, 112

Gouda cheese, sardines with, 126, 129

Gout, 42, 102

Grains, 96

Guanosine diphosphate, 105

Handbook of Diet Therapy (Turner), 102

Hardening of the arteries: Vitamin B$_{15}$ and, 111

Heart disease, 15, 22, 23, 62, 73-75; cholesterol and, 73, 75, 81; diabetes and, 85; "low-fat" diets and, 73-74; nonvertebrate seafoods and, 44; symptoms of, 74, 75, 81

Hendler, Dr. Sheldon S., 7-10, 103

Heparin, 86

Hepatitis, 56

Hero, sardine, 123

Histones, 30

Honey, 92

Hors d'oeuvre, sardine, 122-123

Hydroxyproline, 91

Inositol, 86, 87

Intermittent claudication, 86

Iron, 91

Isoprene, 79-80, 80n

Journal of the American Dietetic Association, 102

Journal of the American Medical Association, 45

Juices, fruits and vegetable, 42, 92, 97

Dell Bestsellers

☐ F.I.S.T. by Joe Eszterhas	$2.25	(12650-9)
☐ ROOTS by Alex Haley	$2.75	(17464-3)
☐ CLOSE ENCOUNTERS OF THE THIRD KIND		
by Steven Spielberg	$1.95	(11433-0)
☐ THE TURNING by Justin Scott	$1.95	(17472-4)
☐ THE CHOIRBOYS by Joseph Wambaugh ...	$2.25	(11188-9)
☐ WITH A VENGEANCE by Gerald DiPego ...	$1.95	(19517-9)
☐ THIN AIR by George E. Simpson		
and Neal R. Burger	$1.95	(18709-5)
☐ BLOOD AND MONEY by Thomas Thompson .	$2.50	(10679-6)
☐ STAR FIRE by Ingo Swann	$1.95	(18219-0)
☐ PROUD BLOOD by Joy Carroll	$1.95	(11562-0)
☐ NOW AND FOREVER by Danielle Steel	$1.95	(11743-7)
☐ IT DIDN'T START WITH WATERGATE		
by Victor Lasky	$2.25	(14400-0)
☐ DEATH SQUAD by Herbert Kastle	$1.95	(13659-8)
☐ DR. FRANK'S NO-AGING DIET		
by Dr. Benjamin S. Frank with Philip Miele ..	$1.95	(11908-1)
☐ SNOWMAN by Norman Bogner	$1.95	(18152-6)
☐ RABID by David Anne	$1.95	(17460-0)
☐ THE SECOND COMING OF LUCAS BROKAW		
by Matthew Braun	$1.95	(18091-0)
☐ THE HIT TEAM by David B. Tinnin		
with Dag Christensen	$1.95	(13644-X)
☐ EYES by Felice Picano	$1.95	(12427-1)
☐ A GOD AGAINST THE GODS		
by Allen Drury	$1.95	(12968-0)
☐ RETURN TO THEBES by Allen Drury	$1.95	(17296-9)
☐ THE HITE REPORT by Shere Hite	$2.75	(13690-3)
☐ THE OTHER SIDE OF MIDNIGHT		
by Sidney Sheldon	$1.95	(16067-7)

At your local bookstore or use this handy coupon for ordering:

DELL BOOKS
P.O. BOX 1000, PINEBROOK, N.J. 07058

Please send me the books I have checked above. I am enclosing $_____
(please add 35¢ per copy to cover postage and handling). Send check or money
order—no cash or C.O.D.'s. Please allow up to 8 weeks for shipment.

Mr/Mrs/Miss_____

Address_____

City_____ State/Zip_____

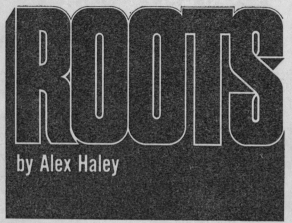

*A rending story of
the power of love*

Now and Forever

Danielle Steel

author of *Passion's Promise*

In one reckless afternoon of passion, Ian had
shattered Jessica's illusion of their perfect
marriage, and Jessica's bitter taunts were driving
them further apart. Faced with the cruelest
separation a man and a woman can know, Jessica
found that reality can be frightening—or
beautiful.

A DELL BOOK $1.95

IN 1918 AMERICA FACED AN ENERGY CRISIS

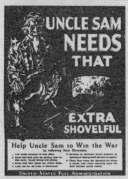

An icy winter gripped the nation. Frozen harbors blocked the movement of coal. Businesses and factories closed. Homes went without heat. Prices skyrocketed. It was America's first energy crisis now long since forgotten, like the winter of '76-'77 and the oil embargo of '73-'74. Unfortunately, forgetting a crisis doesn't solve the problems that cause it. Today, the country is relying too heavily on foreign oil. That reliance is costing us over $40 billion dollars a year Unless we conserve, the world will soon run out of oil, if we don't run out of money first. So the crises of the past may be forgotten, but the energy problems of today and tomorrow remain to be solved. The best solution is the simplest conservation. It's something every American can do.

ENERGY CONSERVATION -
IT'S YOUR CHANCE TO SAVE, AMERICA
Department of Energy, Washington, D.C